Laugh, Sing, and Eat Like a Pig

How an empowered patient beat stage IV cancer (and what healthcare can learn from it)

By "e-Patient Dave" deBronkart

Changing Outlook Press
Media, Pennsylvania

We welcome your comments and suggestions.
Please send them to:
Changing Outlook Press
437 East Franklin Street
Media, PA 19063

or email them to:
george@changingoutlook.com

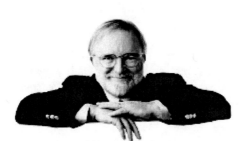

To Tom Ferguson MD
1944-2006
Editor of the medical section of the
Whole Earth Catalog ("Access to Tools")
Visionary founder of the
e-Patient Scholars Working Group

I never met, you,
but you guide me every day

A Note About Treatments

This is a story of a remarkable recovery
by one patient (me)
who received a particular treatment.
That doesn't mean every patient should have what I had;
treatment options are constantly evolving.
If I walked in today,
I might not get the same treatment.

Rather, this is about the power of attitude,
and how e-patients are learning
to be empowered and engaged in their care,
active partners with their care team
in what's being called Participatory Medicine.

An Appeal

Kidney cancer needs to have
more treatments developed.
I encourage patients to inquire
about being in a clinical trial, as I was:
it's only through research
that we can make progress against this disease.

Trials may or may not be available
at your local cancer center,
but you may feel it's worth traveling
to explore your options.
I would have, if necessary.

Thank you!

Contents

Three Introductory Essays

How do you introduce a book that has so many dimensions? Three visionaries who I consider close friends or advisors all agreed to write an introduction, or foreword, or preface ... they're all essays, and I decided to present them here in chronological order of their influence on my experience.

Daniel Z. Sands, MD, MPH
Dave's primary care physician since 2003

Paul F. Levy
President and CEO of Dave's hospital

Matthew Holt
Founder, The Health Care Blog

◆ ◆ ◆

Putting Information — and Knowledge — in Patients' Hands

By Daniel Z. Sands, MD, MPH

*Senior Medical Informatics Director,
Cisco Internet Business Solutions Group
Attending Physician,
Beth Israel Deaconess Medical Center
(Dave's primary care physician since 2003)*

"Knowledge is Power," wrote Francis Bacon. Nowhere is that more true than in healthcare. Knowledge allows us to care for and advocate for our health most effectively. This is especially true in chronic and serious illness.

It is said that information is a prerequisite for knowledge (and

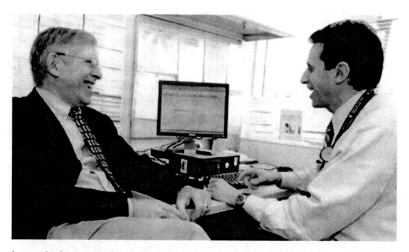

knowledge, combined with insight and experience, can lead to wisdom), and yet physicians often avoid sharing information with patients. This information asymmetry causes patients to be deprived of the tools they need to care for themselves.

Why the reason for this asymmetry? Physicians and patients have historically played roles, with the physician as oracle of knowledge and high priest and the patient as helpless supplicant, desperately appealing to the physician for help in channeling a cure to the patient. Many (perhaps most) physicians cling to that model in some form. They are comfortable in the role as the expert, enjoy the power that comes with knowledge, and are therefore hesitant to share information with patients. Moreover, they often bristle when patients take it upon themselves to learn about their conditions, or ask about things they have read online or in the popular media. And heaven forbid they want to review their own medical records!

In defense of physicians, they spent many years in study and forced learning of facts. Sharing this information without appropriate context not only devalues their hard work but may mislead the patient. Moreover, as physician reimbursement is ever declining, time spent educating patients—which is not generally reimbursed—is time taken away from generating revenue. Whatever the reasons, it is often difficult for patients to find physicians with whom they can partner in a mutually respectful and meaningful way, which includes full information sharing.

While this model may have been appropriate in the pre-scientific era of medicine, it no longer serves us well. We know that knowledgeable, engaged patients can more effectively care for themselves and partner with their physicians, leading to better health outcomes, more efficient healthcare, and improved satisfaction for all involved.

What are types of information that can help patients? They fall into three classes based on their availability to patients. Each patient is already an expert on certain types of information, such as about their own bodies, living situation, and how they manage their health today. Others, such as information about specific diseases or the latest medical literature, were previously the tightly guarded domain of physicians, but are newly available to everyone thanks to the democratizing effect of the Internet. The last bastion of restricted information has been — ironically — information about what lies in that patient's own medical record.

Enlightened healthcare institutions, including Beth Israel Deaconess Medical Center, where Dave gets his care and I practice, are trying to make all information available to patients. This institution has a long history of putting patients first, including promulgating one of the first Patient Bill of Rights in the 1970s. We and other like-minded believe that informed patients make better healthcare decisions and are better partners in their healthcare. In 2000 we were one of the first US medical centers to make patients' records available online through PatientSite, which Dave used to obtain his personal health information. I believe that all patients should have the right to view their medical records online whenever they wish.

But even with this information, it must be transformed into knowledge for it to be powerful. Physicians, nurses, and health educators can help with this, but patients increasingly help each other, through online communities. In these communities, such as ACOR (which Dave used on my recommendation), have mature and robust communities that help countless patients and caregivers with various forms of cancer. All patients facing serious illness should avail themselves of these communities.

So we see how information is increasingly available, and how it can be transformed into knowledge. This should result, as Francis Bacon wrote, in power. However, the real power in the physician-patient relationship comes from both parties sharing information and ideas freely, in an engaged, participatory, and mutually respectful environment. Both the patient and the physician benefit from this, and this power is greater than the power that each participant had on his own.

♦   ♦   ♦

Yes, Patients *Can* Help Their Doctors

By Paul F. Levy, *President and CEO, Beth Israel Deaconess Medical Center, Boston, Massachusetts*

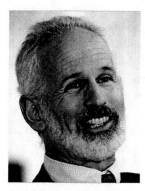

In early January, 2007, Dave deBronkart called to tell me he had stage four renal cancer, and that his life expectancy was 5.5 months. I was chairing our MIT '72 class reunion that year. I said, "Dave, that doesn't work. We need you at the event in June."

A little bad humor was all I could offer at that moment. Later, I found that my hospital, Beth Israel Deaconess Medical Center, could offer much more. We had advanced treatments for Dave's disease. As explained in his story here, those treatments worked very well. He not only made it to the class reunion, but he is still around to write this book.

But the treatment is not the real theme of the book. The theme is the journey of patient empowerment that Dave led for his own sake. And the real story is what Dave taught our doctors and nurses, and what he is now helping to teach the entire country, as he has become one of the nation's leaders in this arena.

The standard view of the medical profession with regard to patient involvement in managing their illness is that "an informed patient will be more compliant with the regimens we say are necessary." In other words, the information goes in one direction: We are the experts. We'll answer your questions. But we are the experts.

I suppose we could spend a long time discussing the sociological reasons for this view. Medical people have always been highly revered in society. They go through intense technical training and have a broad scientific understanding of the human body and its diseases. They are trained, too, to be decisive, using the evidence at hand to make clinical decisions in real time. They are told that part of their job is to not make mistakes and that they have ultimate responsibility for the welfare of their patients.

Given this background, how would we ever expect a doctor to expect that a patient has something to offer in determining the path for clinical treatment of a complex disease like cancer, or even simpler medical problems?

But the truth is that the patients can bring a lot to the party. Let's explore why. First, an MD's knowledge of any given disease is incomplete. With the rapid pace of medical discovery, it is virtually impossible for a doctor to be up to date with everything going on. Second, we need to admit that doctors generally do not practice evidence-based medicine. Experts like Intermountain Health's Brent James have pointed out the high degree in variability with which virtually identical patients are treated. He uses terms like "regional medical mythology" in describing this lack of standardization.

But there is another factor to consider as well. Even if doctors can keep up with the latest scientific information and even if they assiduously try to apply it, the degree of variability among patients themselves makes it difficult to assume that the general statistics (think 5.5 months) apply to the particular case. Any probability distribution is, in fact, a distribution with tails (aka "outliers.") One that is based on a relatively small number of cases is particularly subject to wide standard deviations. One that is based on emerging treatment technologies and approaches is even more subject to a lack of specificity. In short, a problem in medicine is that a statistic often gives the impression of precision when precision is lacking.

In this situation, there is another source of information for the doctor, someone who has an intense vested interest in success — the patient. Now, let's admit that Dave was an outlier himself when it came to patient involvement. He is computer savvy and was indefatigable (yes, even with cancer) in searching out the latest about everything.

But, as I have talked with dozens of other patients, it is apparent that they spend a lot of time exploring the web, participating in support groups, and talking with friends and families about their medical situations. When I have talked with doctors here, they are replete with stories about how a patient has helped them resolve difficult treatment decisions. Sometimes this happens because of technical information provided by patients. Often, though, it is because the patient has "inside" information about his or her own body that puts the doctor's technical knowledge into a more immediate and precise context.

Dave's story offers a dramatic exposition of the advances in cancer treatment that can turn an acutely fatal outcome into a long life. His more important story is how doctors and a patient working in partnership can learn from one another. His plan is to shift the balance of power in clinical settings into a true balance of power, one based on mutual knowledge, respect, and empathy.

I, for one, am glad that he was able to attend that reunion.

♦   ♦   ♦

Changing Relationships and Changing Technology

By Matthew Holt, *Founder, The Health Care Blog*

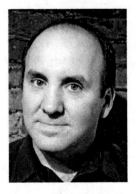

There's a lot that's unusual about Dave's story – today. The interesting question is, what will make the best parts of this story commonplace?

There are two factors. One's moving along fast, another isn't.

The first is a key change in the doctor-patient relationship: participation. The easier availability of more information gives patients a chance to work better with their physicians – to be better educated, which lets the physician have a better time of it. Patients can have a better understanding of what their role is in their outcome. Dave got it in part by other patients helping to target his search; others are getting it from tracking their own personal health information. In any case patients today can know a lot more than a generation ago. And it's already much easier than when Dave was sick in 2007. This part is moving fast.

The second factor is coming, but not as fast as it should: better connectivity. Dave had online messaging with his physician, and someday everyone will, with better record keeping as part of it. For the same reason better coordination between physicians is coming. Most records are still on paper, and tests get redone needlessly, but we're starting to see sharing of tests, images and more getting easier for clinicians.

It's not here yet but we can taste the fact that better information for the physician and the patient makes getting to the right decision easier.

Prolog: Four Early Lessons in Patient Empowerment

When I left college, Nixon was president and I was a hippie. The Vietnam war was raging, and I was in Cambridge – a major center of hippie thinking.

Not that I was doing much thinking, if you know what I mean.

One evening I visited a dentist in Inman Square, a recent graduate of Tufts Medical School. He did something nobody'd ever done: told me, straight up, what my choices were.

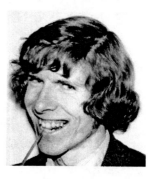

"You can keep caring for your mouth the way you've been, and some years from now, your teeth will fall out." (Like many hippies of the day, I was not subject to the tyranny of bathing.) "Or you can take care of them, and they'll last longer." It was completely clear, with no right or wrong, that it was my choice.

Lesson 1: It's up to me.

◆   ◆   ◆

Five years later I had a small skin cancer (basal cell carcinoma) on my nose, so I was referred to a plastic surgeon. I felt uncomfortable at check-in when I had to sign a waiver of liability *for his corporation,* promising not to sue them no matter what, before I could talk to him.

I felt more uncomfortable when, being a *Consumer Reports* reader, I asked questions, and he didn't like it. Especially when I asked if there would be a scar: he huffed up and said "I *am* a plastic surgeon" in an unpleasant tone.

Well, he taught me who's the doctor: for a 4mm (1/6") lesion, he took a 1/2" flap of skin from my cheek and swung it up over the nostril, without even trying to disguise it: today I have a 1/2" bubble on my nose.

He never came to see me in the hospital – I even had to check myself out. A year later he skipped town to Florida amid rumors of an ethics investigation.

Lesson 2: When your instincts say scram, scram.

◆　　◆　　◆

In the 1990s I had a great periodontist several towns away. Because of the distance I left him in favor of a closer one. But the new guy gave me the creeps: as he was examining my teeth, counting off numbers for his assistant to record, I felt like he was anticipating a new BMW. (I actually imagined a BMW logo reflected in his glasses.)

Remembering the plastic surgeon, this time I spoke up: "I'm really not feeling comfortable—I'm feeling hurried." He backed off apologetically and said we could stop, and I could come back another time. I thanked them and left.

But on the way out, the office wanted payment anyway: "You can come back, but that will be another appointment." "For another charge??" "Yes, of course."

Of course, I didn't come back. And a year later I heard he'd been deported to Ireland for tax evasion.

Lesson 3: If they think your feelings are your problem, you might want to find someone else.

Lesson 4: It's worth traveling to find a doctor you work well with.

E-Patient Precedents

This book is about e-patients. Empowered, Engaged, Equipped, Enabled, Educated … e-patients are effective partners with their clinicians, practicing what we now call "participatory medicine":

> Participatory Medicine is a movement in which networked patients shift from being mere passengers to responsible drivers of their health, and in which providers encourage and value them as full partners.
>
> — Society for Participatory Medicine, April 2010

E-patients gained national notoriety in 2009, but the movement has deep roots.

- When I was just out of college, in Boston, a media uproar arose about a book that told women they could learn about their "female parts" in ways that previously were simply not discussed. That book was *Our Bodies, Ourselves*, and it found a lasting audience: it's in its twelfth edition, with the thirteenth due in 2011.

- A generation earlier, in 1946, Dr. Benjamin Spock's *Baby and Child Care* opened with this advice to parents: "Trust yourself. You know more than you think you do."

It turns out that given a chance, people like to know how their bodies work. And many like to be active in healthcare – especially when something goes wrong.

Chapter 1: The first four weeks (and where the title comes from)

My online posts (which are the basis for most of this book) started on January 30, 2007, on my CaringBridge journal. But the story starts four weeks earlier, when I got an x-ray for a simple shoulder problem, and it showed a mass that turned out to be a metastatic tumor from kidney cancer. Now, if you think back to four weeks ago today (as you read this), it probably doesn't seem like long ago. But in those four weeks my world turned upside down and inside out, so much that when I started working on this book, I was dismayed to find that some CaringBridge messages were apparently lost. It turns out the reason was simple: all those messages had been written before the CaringBridge journal started, during those first four weeks.

It's amazing how much my perspective on life altered during those weeks—it's as if my life's memories suddenly had a new starting point and everything was referenced from there. It rather reminds me of the often-reported experience of realizing you're about to be in a car accident and discovering that your mind suddenly goes into slow motion. (That happened to me when I was a passenger in an accident when I was 16. Eerie.)

The messages I'd sought were the original communications from which the title of the book arose. In those first days my extraordinary family members and I whirled into action, looking for resources, every single thing we could get our hands on. See, all the data I could find online about my form of cancer said things like "prognosis is grim" or "outlook is poor." With those odds, I very quickly took inventory of what was available, particularly in the mind-body arena.

We quickly planned to have me (and wife Ginny) attend one of the "Exceptional Cancer Patient" retreats co-developed by Dr. Bernie Siegel. Another resource I'd long known about was the curative power of laughter as famously described by *Saturday Review* editor Norman Cousins in *Anatomy of an Illness*, recounting that belly-laughing to Marx Brothers movies served as an anesthetic and, with other mental processes (love, hope, faith), brought him back to health—from incurable disease.

The introduction to *Anatomy* begins:

> The basic theme of this book is that every person must accept a certain measure of responsibility for his or her own recovery from disease or disability.

I certainly agree with those words, although I had never seen them at the time of my healthcare adventures! Yet a year ago I vowed (as if my life depended on it!) to do everything I could to take responsibility for my own outcome. And if that meant laughing my butt off, so be it—it's tough work, but someone's gotta do it!

A while later, as I began rearranging life to adjust to my dwindling energy levels, I discussed options with my primary physician, Dr. Danny Sands. I have an active singing hobby, participating with a great group of men in the Nashua, NH chapter of the Barbershop Harmony Society, nee SPEBSQSA. I told Dr. Sands I was considering dropping that activity, and he said no. "You do not want to start dropping life activities that you love," he wisely said. "It sends the wrong signal. Plus, the oxygen exchange will do you good for what lies ahead."

Well, cool, I thought—laugh and sing! I can deal with that.

The corker came in late January, when I got instructions on preparing my body for the physical war that was about to take place, as the cancer kept taking away my body weight and we prepared to fight back, biologically. A hospital nutritionist sent me a diet from the Bizarro planet: How to Increase Your Caloric Intake. It recommended putting whipped cream (real whipped cream) on all desserts, using full-strength pizza for a snack, using whole milk instead of skim. Insane things like that.

"Well," I says to myself, "we might as well have fun with this! Now it's 'laugh, sing, and eat like a pig!'" And, I actually said to myself, "If I ever write a book about this, that's what I'll call it."

2

So here we are. I no longer get to eat whatever I want, but I'm still laughing and singing as much as I can—with an enhanced collection of comedy DVDs, thanks to the generosity of friends and family this past year.

You know, at the start of this adventure, I really did not know how many months of life I had left. I did know I was going to do everything in my power to beat the cancer, whatever that might be. I also knew that whatever time I had left, I was going to live it like crazy ... to laugh, sing, and eat like a pig.

I challenge you to be fully alive, every moment that you have left in life. As you read this book, please listen for how you can face every moment with power and grace, no matter what your circumstance. Take responsibilty for your own life.

So, how perfect is this? While researching Norman Cousins, I ran across this quote:

> "Death is not the greatest loss in life. The greatest loss is what dies inside us while we live."

Amen. No matter what your situation, no matter what your outcome, my most fervent wish is that you be fully alive for every moment you live. That's the essence of the story you're about to read.

Chapter 2: "There's something in your lung"

January 2 – March 5, 2007

On January 2, 2007, a routine shoulder x-ray showed a mass in a nearby part of my lung.

The X-ray that started it all. I had the x-ray because of a rotator cuff problem, but the doctor noticed a nearby mass in my lung.

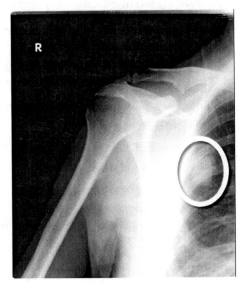

The next day the doc called and said the shoulder would be fine, but they had found a spot on my lung, and I should come back in for a CT scan. They didn't know what it was, he said – "could be a fungus for all we know."

The next week he called and said it was a tumor, and there were "lots of them." I later learned "lots" meant five – but in assessing the prognosis, there are two conditions that matter: either you have one or none, or you have more than that, which worsens the prognosis. So five is "lots," for that purpose.

Apparently they were in both lungs. (I keep thinking how lucky I am to have no symptoms!) He said they did look like cancer but not lung cancer – something blood-borne from somewhere

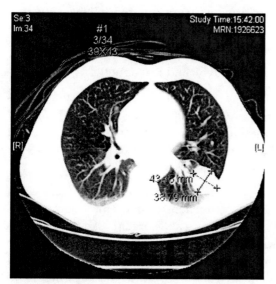

First CT scan shows a big tumor (lower right). The lines with x's show its dimensions.

else. Next step: get an abdominal ultrasound. Thursday 1/11 my wife Ginny came along (she's watched ultrasounds as a vet) and we saw it: a darker mass in the right kidney. A CT scan that night confirmed it.

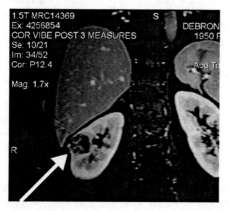

Primary tumor. A sizeable chunk of my right kidney had been displaced by cancer.

That night was hell. My online research said that the median survival time for metastasized kidney cancer, with my prognostic factors, is 5.5 months. Never see another Christmas? Maybe not even see summer??

I later learned that's a very misleading statistic, based mostly on data collected when treatments were not as effective. But that night I didn't know it. I awoke at 1 AM, and could not get back to sleep – I was possessed by the implications.

I continued losing weight, slowly, and lost appetite.

A note about this pattern of "kidney to lung": The kidney filters blood, which then goes directly to the heart, where it's pumped at full strength into the lungs. If a kidney cancer drops a nasty pellet in the blood, it gets stuck at the first tight place it finds – the capillaries in the lung.

After the shock passed, a major turnaround happened when my MD referred me to an excellent online email community, the kidney cancer list at www.ACOR.org. (I like to say "My doctor prescribed ACOR," because he literally wrote it on a slip of paper and handed it to me.) I learned a lot from patients and caregivers who are very actively involved in the latest info, and I got empowered to get my buns in gear, learning and getting in action.

◆   ◆   ◆

From here on, almost all of this book is based on entries I posted online. Initially, these were made in CaringBridge (www. caringbridge.org), a free service which allows patients to keep their loved ones up to date on their medical condition. Later, I started a blog of my own and posted material there.

Monday, January 29, 2007 10:11 PM

News so good, we went to the Cheesecake Factory!

First visit to the oncologist! Today, in a 2-1/2 hour visit to Beth Israel Deaconess Medical Center ("BIDMC," formed from Beth Israel Hospital and Deaconess Medical Center), Ginny and I

Note about links to the Web

By the time you read this book, websites may have changed. Up-to-date versions of all links (URLs) mentioned in this book can be found on this book's website at www.laughsingbook.com/links.

6

met the oncologist, and the urologist/surgeon who'll take out my kidney, and an oncology Fellow, and the nurse who runs the clinical trial I'll be in. We got updates on everything. We heard many things that improved our view beyond what we'd already learned. By the end, we felt so uplifted we went to dinner at the Cheesecake Factory!

Here's a summary of what we learned and what's next:

- We expect that my offending kidney will be removed in late February. [Update: the date was moved to 3/19, then back to 3/6.] It's now possible to do this via laparoscopy, with a few small incisions (2-3 weeks to recover) instead of a big 8 inch incision (2-3 *months* to recover). Once that's done, the next stage of treatment can be chosen and begin.

- At this hospital, HDIL-2 (high dosage Interleukin 2) therapy apparently goes better than at most. [There's more information about HDIL-2 in the next post.] I'd read that it's effective in a small number of cases: 7%, 13%, or 20%, depending on whose study you read. At BIDMC they get 20% response.

- Unlike most places, BIDMC has (as mentioned earlier) gotten good enough at HDIL-2 that it doesn't require being in the ICU: you stay in a special unit, where they can manage the cases well enough that ICU is no longer necessary.

- They also offer low-dosage Interleukin, but the HDIL now works well enough that they always recommend it first, for patients who are well qualified (in terms of strength and disease state). I'm well qualified.

- People who do respond to HDIL tend to have lasting responses. (If the tumor disappears, it tends to stay gone; if it shrinks, it tends to stay shrunk.) This is a huge breakthrough, considering that less than ten years ago kidney cancer had nothing that resembled a cure.

- They have a new experimental treatment, a tumor vaccine, that's much more gentle than any of the established treatments, which all have significant possible side effects.

- They want one more scan (an MRI) to confirm the diagnosis.

They'll scan the kidneys, and also the brain, to confirm that there are no brain mets (metastases). That's probably Tuesday (tomorrow). Then a team of 20 docs assesses my case, at their weekly Thursday meeting (2/1 or 2/8).

- Next meeting with the docs is probably Monday 2/12. Meanwhile, I love the flyer the nutritionist mailed me: "How to increase your caloric intake." (Yes, increase.) It includes such tips as using whole milk instead of 2%, putting real whipped cream on all desserts, eating ice cream, using butter instead of margarine, etc.

We are more optimistic than ever.

Tuesday, January 30, 2007 9:32 PM

Today I had my MRI, and (separately) they set the date for the nephrectomy (kidney removal): Monday, March 19. If all goes as planned I'll be back home 3/21.

My next event will be the next meeting with the doctors, probably Monday 2/12.

The March 19 nephrectomy date means I'll be able to sing at my chorus's spring competition the weekend of March 17. Yay!

Tuesday, January 30, 2007 10:44 PM

Several people have asked about the "HDIL-2" treatment I mentioned. Here's a description compiled from what I've learned.

HDIL-2 is high dosage Interleukin-2. It's the only thing that's been known to produce a cure for RCC (renal cell carcinoma) – actually the docs are more cautious – they'll only call it a "persistent complete response." (Tumors are gone and stay gone for 10 years or more.) Sounds good to me!

Interleukin-2 has long been given in low dosages (ordinary regular treatments). But for about 10 years (maybe longer) it's also been given intensively – high dosage (HDIL-2). The side effects are

The right doctor in the right setting

In the prolog I described four lessons I'd learned earlier in life, which taught me to be responsible for my choice of doctors. Those lessons were at play a few years before cancer struck, as I continued to be proactive in where I got my care.

Getting cured of Stage IV cancer was a miracle, but it was also the result of two choices that had been made years earlier, long before I had any inkling that I would get seriously ill.

My first decision: "It's up to me what kind of doctor I have."

I wanted to make a conscious decision about my care. It's not like putting a quarter in a prize-dispensing machine and taking whatever comes out. Like a self-aware consumer of any service – a shopper – I decided on my priorities. Different providers have different skills and different styles.

My second decision: "I'm going to shop around."

I decided I wanted a doctor who was affiliated with a major teaching hospital. That decision eliminated the doctors and hospitals nearest my home. But my first wife, a nurse, told me, "Whenever it gets dicey, you want someone who handles a lot of cases like yours."

At the first hospital I tried, I found a good doctor, but the rest of the staff seemed disempowered. Frequently, their attitude seemed to be, "That's the way it is; there's nothing I can do." I knew I didn't want that culture if I ever found myself in a life-and-death situation.

So I tried another teaching hospital that I heard had a can-do attitude. I liked what I found there, and I got connected with a marvelous doctor. That doctor and that hospital were ultimately key factors in the care that saved my life.

significant and nasty, which is why it's typically delivered only in ICU. But apparently Beth Israel has the whole protocol tightened down well enough, and has enough experience (about 100 HDIL patients/yr) that they can do it in a special non-intensive-care unit.

You go in Monday, and get the crap beaten out of you medically for 4 days. You recover for 48 hrs, then go home Sunday, continue recovering for a week, then come back in for a second (worse) week. Another week recovering, and you can go back to work when you feel like it. Some weeks later they scan you to see the status of the tumors.

80% of patients don't respond; 20% do. [Updated 2/11/07: Those 20% who do respond tend to have lasting responses (the tumor reduction or disappearance does not go away), and HALF of those who respond have a COMPLETE response – the disease disappears.]

For whatever reason, I'm confident that I'll be in the top group. If I understand correctly, the persistent response means HDIL-2 is the only treatment for which a recurrence a few years down the road is not common.

It would be a bizarre and wild ride to get diagnosed with something that has a median survival time of 5.5 months, yet actually be cured within that timeframe. (Excuse me – actually have a "persistent complete response.")

Thursday, February 1, 2007 10:38 PM,

CHOCOLATE THERAPY!

I'd heard the expression before, but it only dawned on me today that it might be relevant to me.

I got a couple of Hershey bars for Christmas and had been ignoring their existence. This morning my eye lit on them and I realized they fit marvelously into my instructions to increase caloric intake.

This probably isn't what most people have in mind when they talk about chocolate therapy, but it works for me.

♦   ♦   ♦

Tuesday night I had two MRIs. One was of the kidneys, to inform the surgeon who'll remove the offending one. The other was of the brain, to make sure there aren't any brain "mets" (metastases), because I had two very short dizziness episodes in December. The brain MRI came back negative: no problem found.

Saturday, February 3, 2007 10:12 AM

Great news: all the encouragement and feeding tips I've been getting have produced results – I gained 6 pounds this week! This is the most I've weighed since Thanksgiving. Hotcha.

Saturday, February 3, 2007 5:17 PM

The ACOR kidney cancer email list that I read is a fountain of useful information and empowering thought. I want to share with you something I read today, posted by an MD who is himself a kidney cancer patient.

I realized last week that success in this journey doesn't require a complete disappearance of the tumors. (Disappearance is my goal, of course, but I've learned that many people simply stop the disease in its tracks so it never gets worse, or the tumors shrink and stay that way. That would be fine with me: I'd be happy to feel this way for the next 20-30 years!)

And today I discovered that I'm not the only one thinking that way – there may be a shift occurring within the cancer care community. Here's what the MD posted:

> "I do think that there is a paradigm change occurring in cancer treatment. In the past all anyone wanted to see was a shrinkage in tumor size – whether in a test mouse or a patient. This is still used and is often how a med gets FDA approved. Unfortunately this often does not translate to real improvement in the patient's outcome – in whether they survive longer and with fewer symptoms.

> "Now people are starting to talk about looking at how treatment prolongs the time that patients show *no change* in their tumors (PFS – progression free survival) and how long they live with their cancer (OS – overall survival). So cancer is being looked at as a chronic disease, much like diabetes, asthma, congestive heart failure, etc."

"ACOR was invaluable"

The ACOR community was invaluable. They helped with interpreting what the docs were saying. They helped him set expectations for treatment.   – Dave's wife Ginny

11

Another list member commented later: "I have had my thinking adjusted 180 degrees by the idea that this can be a long term chronic thing, not a death sentence."

As I say, having it stay this way would be fine with me. I'm still going for the big Kahuna, but the landscape of possible "We win!" outcomes is much bigger than it was when I first read those "median survival time" statistics.

This exemplifies that one of the most important things I've learned in the past month is to keep thinking for myself and keep asking questions.

♦   ♦   ♦

The Seven Preliminary Conclusions

It's early in the story but I'd like to introduce a remarkable document that I discovered a year later: "The e-Patients White Paper." You'll hear more later in this book, but here's a taste, from Chapter 2 of the paper. See Appendix A for more information.

1. e-Patients have become valuable contributors, and providers should recognize them as such.

"When clinicians acknowledge and support their patients' role in self-management ... they exhibit fewer symptoms, demonstrate better outcomes, and require less professional care."

2. The art of empowering patients is trickier than we thought.

"We now know that empowering patients requires a change in their level of engagement, and in the absence of such changes, clinician-provided [information] has few, if any, positive effects."

3. We have underestimated patients' ability to provide useful online resources.

Fabulous story of the "best of the best" web sites for mental health, as determined by a doctor in that field without considering who runs each site. Of the sixteen sites, ten were produced by patients, five by professionals, and one by a bunch of artists and researchers at Xerox PARC!

4. We have overestimated the hazards of imperfect online health information.

An eye-opener: in four years of looking for "death by googling," even with a fifty-euro bounty for each reported death(!), Dr. Gunther Eysenbach (now head of the Journal of Medical Internet Research) found only one possible case.

One more note: Ginny and daughter Lindsey and I went to D.C. to hear my sister Suede perform. It was a moving experience – something shifted for me during Suede's performance of "Never Never Land." (There is a video on YouTube of Suede singing this song.) It was a transformational moment: I suddenly got something, and my view of the world shifted. I'd been fatigued that afternoon, but I went out with Suede until 1 a.m. and I had no fatigue at all this week (until Friday afternoon), and I'm fine today.

Saturday we got together with the siblings who are local, and that too was rejuvenating.

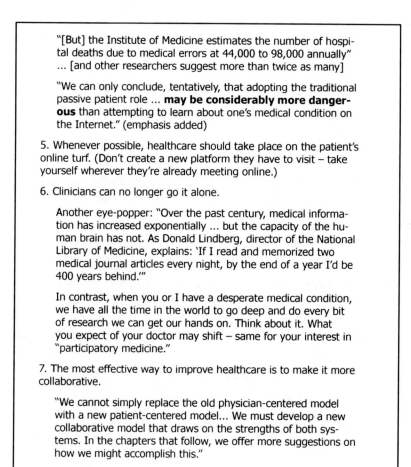

"[But] the Institute of Medicine estimates the number of hospital deaths due to medical errors at 44,000 to 98,000 annually" ... [and other researchers suggest more than twice as many]

"We can only conclude, tentatively, that adopting the traditional passive patient role ... **may be considerably more dangerous** than attempting to learn about one's medical condition on the Internet." (emphasis added)

5. Whenever possible, healthcare should take place on the patient's online turf. (Don't create a new platform they have to visit – take yourself wherever they're already meeting online.)

6. Clinicians can no longer go it alone.

Another eye-popper: "Over the past century, medical information has increased exponentially ... but the capacity of the human brain has not. As Donald Lindberg, director of the National Library of Medicine, explains: 'If I read and memorized two medical journal articles every night, by the end of a year I'd be 400 years behind.'"

In contrast, when you or I have a desperate medical condition, we have all the time in the world to go deep and do every bit of research we can get our hands on. Think about it. What you expect of your doctor may shift – same for your interest in "participatory medicine."

7. The most effective way to improve healthcare is to make it more collaborative.

"We cannot simply replace the old physician-centered model with a new patient-centered model... We must develop a new collaborative model that draws on the strengths of both systems. In the chapters that follow, we offer more suggestions on how we might accomplish this."

How many things can *you* stay expert at?

According to Paul Grundy, MD, Director of Worldwide Health Operations for IBM, the average physician's practice needs a customer base (a "panel," they call it) of 1500-2000 patients to make ends meet.

Think about that: roughly speaking, that means for every "one in a thousand" disease, each physician has one or two patients! Who could keep up with the latest on every one-in-a-thousand disease?

In contrast to this, a community of patients like my ACOR kidney cancer group is focused on just one thing: kidney cancer. That's one of the key reasons why communities of e-patients can truly help physicians – a cornerstone of participatory medicine.

Suede is an amazing person – generous, deeply into nurturing and spiritual energy, and a deeply soulful jazz and blues singer.

Tuesday, February 6, 2007 9:52 PM

My surgery date has been moved up to March 6, which is fine with me! Git that thing outa me!

♦   ♦   ♦

Today I learned of two web sites that provide other services for patients and their families:

http://www.lotsahelpinghands.com/ is a group calendar that patients' families can use to coordinate assistance from friends & families – things like arranging rides, bringing meals over, etc.

http://CarePages.com/ is more like CaringBridge. "CarePages are free, personal, private web pages that help family and friends communicate when someone is facing illness." Isn't it wonderful that caring people out there are making services like this available?

♦   ♦   ♦

As many of you know, my hospital (Beth Israel Deaconess) has a wonderful secure patient web site, PatientSite, where my medical records are visible to me, including CAT scan and MRI reports, and I can send and receive secure emails with the physicians. It's an incredibly open process, which really relieves me of wondering "what they know that I don't know."

Last summer I sent a note to the doc updating him on my blood pressure, and the next thing I heard, he'd electronically sent a prescription change to my nearby Walgreen's, and it was ready to pick up. No need to get a call back from the doctor, etc. And since it's secure email inside their system, it's outside the reach of Internet snoopers.

But that freedom brings responsibility: if you choose to look into that section, you have be careful about what you read – just as if you were opening your folder in the doctor's office. I got scared (briefly) about something I read this weekend, left an email for my oncologist, and got it cleared up.

Of course that also requires doctors who are very open – it requires two-way trust and open communication, and willingness to take what may be a lot of questions between appointments.

◆　　◆　　◆

Kendra Bradley is the nurse who coordinates the HDIL-2 program that I'll probably be in. Tonight I called to say I asked my email group to send me their stories about the side effects they experienced, because I like to know what to expect before I do something new.

Would you do it for your child? Then do it for yourself.

One of the best points I learned in 11 years in pediatric bone marrow transplant is that parents tend to have more freedom to advocate for their child. When one moves over to adult medicine, it suddenly seems like advocating for a family member or for oneself is perceived as 'less acceptable'.

No parent would have their child cared for without asking questions and getting information. Why would that be the slightest bit different in the adult setting? In fact, it is critical to recognize the parents as the "expert" on their own child or the adult patient as the "expert" on themselves.

– Kendra Bradley, research coordinator for my clinical trial

I told her I'm that kinda guy, and she said, in a strong confident voice, "I knew that." I said "You did?" She said "I had you pegged five minutes into our first visit." We liked her immediately on that first visit, so this kind of thing is another confidence builder.

So I'm going to paste all the HDIL-2 stories into a Word document for her to read at her convenience, so she can comment on whether it sounds pretty accurate for how it goes at Beth Israel Deaconess. See, I intend to be prepared when I go in there.

'Night!

Friday, February 9, 2007 12:16 AM

I'm gonna be on PBS! And it has nothing to do with cancer. How's that??

They're flying me to D.C. next Tuesday, where the local PBS station is filming a pilot program "that explores the scope of the health care quality challenge facing America and the promise of health information technology for quality improvement. ... the 60-minute pilot program will discuss in-depth how health information technology is changing health care in America. The program will be hosted by Frank Sesno, contributing CNN correspondent and Professor of Communications at George Washington University."

I'll be on a panel (with two MDs and a nurse!) during the segment that discusses solutions. I'll be talking about my hospital's PatientSite system.

What a life I have.

♦   ♦   ♦

Thank you so much to all the new visitors, for all your supportive words in the Guestbook. I can hardly express how it feels to have so many people out there pulling for me.

♦   ♦   ♦

Today I signed up to be a walker in the Avon breast cancer walk, which is May 19-20 in Boston. A key factor is that training for it

16

will give me a local community that supports me in EXERCISING! That's something the doctor told me to do, which doesn't come nearly as easily as the "eat like a pig" part.

Saturday, February 10, 2007 7:53 PM

MEDICAL UPDATE

Weekly Saturday morning weigh-in: Gained another 3 pounds. That's 9 total since I got the instructions to bulk up.

◆ ◆ ◆

My case was reviewed Thursday by the hospital's tumor board, and Monday afternoon is when we find out their treatment plan. Then I fly to DC for the PBS thing on Tuesday. More news Monday night when I get to the hotel.

That's all the medical news for now. Below is some chit-chat. Thanks for tuning in.

◆ ◆ ◆

I'm visiting Mom again in Maryland this weekend, with the ultimate purpose of seeing niece Becky (13) play the mayor's wife in The Music Man tomorrow. Nothin' like a Broadway smash with barbershop singin'!

Monday, February 12, 2007 11:26 PM

We met tonight with the oncologist and the HDIL-2 nurse. Kidney surgery is confirmed for 3/6/07.

The HDIL-2 treatment can begin earlier than I thought! We may start it April 2 or even March 26.

Several people have asked why we're waiting so long to remove the kidney. The answer is that there are plenty of docs who can do it right away with the "big cut" method, but only one who can do it laparoscopically, which requires just 2-3 weeks to recover. I'm happy to wait a few weeks to cut 2 months off recovery time. :)

[Ginny and I agreed about declining the new experimental

vaccine treatment because it would delay the start of HDIL by several months. This is a very early clinical trial – Phase 1, they call it – and there's just not enough reason for me to postpone the better-known treatment.]

Meanwhile I finally have two physical complaints to grouse about, but they apparently have nothing to do with cancer. (1) My knee has been annoying me for 12 days in various ways, and this weekend got bad enough that today I used a cane; (2) my left forearm is being a pain. (Sister Amy the physical therapist suspects tennis elbow.) They had me get x-rays tonight just to be sure they're not cancer-related.

I would be very happy to go back to the painfree state where all I had was cancer!

Wednesday, February 14, 2007 7:09 PM

MEDICAL UPDATE:

Not what I'd hoped. Today we got the results of Monday's x-rays. It does look like the pain in the left knee is a "bone met" – the cancer has metastasized to the left femur (thigh). Rats.

BUT, the surface of the bone is intact, which is good.

Treatment: in the next two weeks they'll zap the femur with radiation. It'll involve a series of visits. I'll also get the bone scan that they'd said we would do if needed. (Now it's needed!)

The forearm x-ray is inconclusive – some deterioration which may or may not be another met. The bone scan will tell more.

Plans for the scheduled kidney removal are unaffected.

If a bone scan shows that there are other mets, then the doc says they'll assess stabilizing them, which may delay the start of HDIL. He reiterated that my case is so new (this all started just 5 weeks ago!) that they have almost no history on me, and they definitely want a clear sense of what body they'd be attacking with this HDIL treatment. I support that approach!

And if HDIL is delayed, then I may go ahead with the experimental vaccine (a Phase I study), which might produce a cure with very little attack to the body. My only reason for saying no to it was that it would have postponed the HDIL.

◆　◆　◆

TELEVISION STAR UPDATE: More than I'd hoped!

Yesterday I had WAY too much fun being videotaped at WETA-TV in D.C. MAN did I have fun! All the panelists spent 2-3 hours together in the "green room." (Yes, I got to be in a green room. Woohoo! It wasn't green – it was a plain white room with folding tables, free lunch, and a BIG tv.)

The host, CNN's Frank Sesno, is an incredible pro. His voice is richly resonant – my singer's ear caught that. We did no rehearsing – they don't discuss questions in advance. He just chatted with us to break the ice, and advised us on a few pointers. (My favorite: "The ladies already know this, but men, you too need to keep your knees together.")

So imagine my surprise when my panel got on the set and after the intro 3-minute video clip played, he turned right to me first and said, "Dave, I understand you were recently diagnosed with kidney cancer. Has PatientSite made a difference in that experience?" And we were off and running. (I didn't know we were going to be talking about my cancer!)

It only lasted 12 minutes and then I ran right to the airport (to wait 4 hours before departure). As I left the room, I said to the woman organizing it, "Why YES, I'd be HAPPY to come back and do THAT again!"

I am way looking forward to that show. As I said, it'll air sometime in the spring, which starts March 21. [The program never did air, but it's on YouTube. Search for "Healthcare 360".]

◆　◆　◆

Aphorism of the day: "Be careful what you wish for – you might get it."

Last weekend when my knee was hurting I told people "I'd be happy to go back to just having cancer!" Well, that's what I got!

19

Laugh, Sing, and Eat Like a Pig

(The pain in my leg is cancer.) I shoulda said "go back to just having cancer with no symptoms!"

Sunday, February 18, 2007 11:35 PM

No medical news except that the danged femur issue has my whole left leg tense, which is very uncomfortable.

Next step is this Wednesday: first meeting with the radiation oncologist who will zap that femur tumor. I hope to get the whole-body bone scan the same day.

♦   ♦   ♦

Great birthday weekend! Ginny organized the best birthday party of my life. A slew of friends & family including daughter Lindsey and beau Jon: terrific food; and the ever-shy (not!) Suede pulled a surprise appearance.

Gifts were centered around the Make Dave Laugh campaign, including a 4-DVD set of Looney Tunes cartoons, and (from Lindsey) the entire first season of Saturday Night Live – 8 DVDs! I am more than equipped for my first hospitalization, humorwise.

♦   ♦   ♦

Taking the advice of many of you, I'm supplementing the surgery etc. with acupuncture. Had my first-ever session Saturday. As is apparently common, the first session didn't produce any big breakthrough. Next session is next Saturday.

Saturday, February 24, 2007 12:44 AM

Thursday: Second radiation treatment. Walking was bugging me enough that I picked up a loose wheelchair in the lobby and wheeled myself to the treatment. Felt good!

My friend Dorron arrived with his whole family from Israel, to visit us for the weekend. The codeine was not agreeing with me: made me very very drowsy and didn't help the knee pain. I started having palpably swollen muscles on my thigh. What is this, things getting worse?? The swelling means it's difficult, painful and slow to sit down or get up.

Lindsey and I went to dinner with Dorron and his family. It was a lot of walking, and I started not feeling well. I had no interest in food at all, and as plates were carried past, I started getting grossed out at the sight of food. What is THIS, are things getting worse here, too?? What is this cancer doing to me? Or is it one of the many nausea reactions I've read about involving cancer treatments??

When our food was brought, right under my nose, that was it: I had to get to the men's room fast. Imagine me trying to get on my feet and cane fast and, as fast as possible, work my way to the men's room. What's going on?? Every day in this cancer trip seems to bring something new. So it's one day after another of "What's THIS?? What's happening? Is it trouble?"

In this case, the moment I barfed, I knew it was just a bad lunch, because I felt completely better (except for the knee). But I decided I'd had enough codeine. In addition to the drowsiness, I'd gotten hiccups on and off all day.

Oh, and I got my spiffy new handicapped parking tag. Mind you, I'm not thrilled to be taking on all these signs of sickness, but the leg pain is quite convincing. "Thou shalt not walk more than you HAVE to" is easy to follow, and that includes getting a handicapped tag.

♦   ♦   ♦

Friday: Doctor okayed moving back to the previous medicine. I woke up with the knee feeling fine, but as soon as I got on my feet the bunched-up muscles started causing trouble again. It took me 90 minutes to bathe and dress and get out of the house.

Third radiation treatment. aHA: the radiation guy explains that swollen tissue is a common side effect of leg radiation. The radiation attacks all the tissue. The tumor cells die; the healthy tissue starts repairing itself in a few hours, and starts by becoming swollen. So THAT's what's going on! Immediately my sense of concern shifted. It makes SUCH a difference to know what's going on. I'm no longer facing the questions about the swelling: "What's going on?? Is it trouble? How long is it going to last? Can they do anything about it?"

Now that I know it's a response to the radiation, I know it'll stop in about a week. I can get through that.

New weird symptom: in my right palm, there's a new hard/thick portion right along one of the lines. What's THIS, now???

My self-awareness has grown: I've figured out that the difficult position is the last 20-30 degrees from the leg being fully extended. So I practice keeping the leg fully extended, and standing occasionally.

Went out with Dorron's family again. MUCH better evening! Leg felt so good that I forgot to take the next medicine. (THAT didn't last long.)

And I figured out that the weird thick skin on my palm was simply a callus from leaning on the cane. Another cause for concern laid to rest.

♦   ♦   ♦

Next steps:

Sat. morning: Acupuncture #2; Monday 2/27: meet orthopedic (bone) doctor; full-body bone scan, to check for more bone mets, 4th radiation treatment on the thigh. Tuesday 2/28: pre-op testing (nephrectomy is a week away); 5th (final) radiation treatment. Friday 3/2: two tests to qualify for the HDIL-2 treatment (stress test and pulmonary function). Tuesday 3/6: surgery.

♦   ♦   ♦

Tuesday: quartet practice in the evening... BOY it feels good to sing close harmony again!

The knee keeps causing difficulty, so I bought a cane – a sturdy, collapsible cane. Web research showed that there are many folding canes that can only support up to 220 pounds (approx my weight). The one to get is from Hugo http://www. hugoanywhere. com – up to 550 pounds!

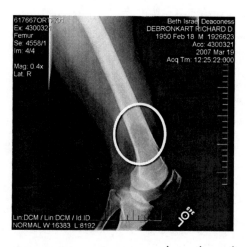

The tumor in my leg.
The slightly dark oval inside the circle is the tumor, which has begun to eat into the surrounding bone.

◆　　◆　　◆

Wednesday: Three doctor's appointments, for the start of radiation treatment. I got a tattoo! Well, the consent form says "I authorize the marking of my skin with tiny permanent marks." I said "You mean a micro-tattoo?" They said "Well, yes." These are to ensure that every radiation treatment is focused on precisely the same spot. Let me just say that the guy who made the marks could learn a few things about gentleness from my acupuncturist.

I guess I'm getting fast-tracked: I had the initial meeting with the radiation doc, the "mapping" session where they x-ray the leg to map out where everything will go, and the first treatment, all in the same day. Four more treatments set for Thursday, Friday, Monday, Tuesday.

I asked to see the original x-ray, and the radiation doc pulled it up on the screen. (I love how open and forthcoming everyone at this hospital is. Don't ever ever tolerate a doc who acts like it's none of your business! Numerous people on the kidney cancer mailing list have reported that defensive docs have too often turned out to also have out-of-date info, sometimes dangerously so.)

In the x-ray I saw the slightly darker area that's the tumor, and saw that there has been some bone erosion from the inside. There's still enough there to be sturdy, which again makes me very happy about that "early detection" shoulder x-ray.

The knee continued to get more painful. Got a prescription to upgrade pain med to Tylenol + Codeine.

Evening: chorus rehearsal. Sat through most of it, but couldn't stand sitting! :) Got on the risers for the last hour; GREAT fun.

Sunday, February 25, 2007 9:24 AM

DEPARTMENT OF TRANSPORTATION

News and views on getting about with a bum knee

Cane findings:

- It's very, very silly to forget where you put it.
- It's hard to find places to prop up a cane where it won't fall over.
- It's not good when it falls on the knee that's painful. I have repeatedly tested this, with consistent results.
- While walking, it's not good when you don't watch where the cane goes, so you kick it. :-)

Motorized grocery scooter learnings:

- These are cool gadgets. They don't go fast but they're reliable, and they turn on a dime.
- Every store seems to have a different model.
- Target Inc. is incredibly stupid. They're only budgeted for two scooters per store! Last Saturday noon, my store had one scooter out and the other one's battery was dead. I saw the other one... the woman trying to drive it was trying to push it, because its battery was dead too.

Wheelchair learnings:

- These are fun, and I'm good at maneuvering them. (I only use them at the hospital.)
- But they're not practical to integrate into my work life. Can't get one into and out of the car by myself.

- I'm not strong enough to get myself up the wheelchair ramp.

Handicapped Parking mirror tags:

- In the N.H. dept of motor vehicles, to get a hang tag you must go to a counter. But that only works if the tag is marked "temporary." If you want a permanent one, you must mail it in to the state capital and wait two weeks.

- If you try to inquire by phoning the registry, you learn that in proudly-no-income-or-sales-tax N.H., they don't have voicemail: you get a busy signal until the line is clear.

- When you actually submit the form in person, for this carefully guarded privileged tag (so no unauthorized tags get into the hands of cheaters), they then ask if you'd like *two*.

It amazes me that all these complications arise from something as seemingly trivial as a bone met, when the primary tumor itself continues to cause no interference with life. This is no small issue because to the cancer docs, a key indicator of outcomes is your "performance factor:" It's very good if your ability to do life functions is unaffected, and your statistical outcome odds get worse when your "performance score" starts to decline.

Sunday, February 25, 2007 11:02 PM

Knee is feeling better today. (No radiation in 2 days, and I stayed off the leg most of the day.) But for tomorrow's back & forth for 4 appointments across BIDMC, I called ahead to arrange transportation.

Tuesday, February 27, 2007 11:17 PM

Very tired tonight, because of two very busy days at the hospital and a half day at work today. Looking forward to a full night's sleep.

Monday I met the orthopedic surgeon (on a "just in case" basis) who will work on my leg in the unlikely event that's necessary.

"The Lethal Lag Time" – and worse

We're raised to only trust medical information that's been published in a peer reviewed journal. A real problem arises because of the time it takes for a completed study to make it into the field.

Chapter 5 of the e-patient white paper calls this "the lethal lag time." It quotes Norman Scherzer, formerly of the Centers for Disease Control and the N.Y. Dept. of Public Health, describing why it takes years for information to make it from the researcher's desk into the hands, eyes, and minds of physicians everywhere. The figure I've heard repeatedly is 2-5 years.

In high tech this effect is called "latency" – the information is out there but hasn't reached us yet. (A common latency experience is if you click something on a website and it takes forever to reach your screen. Latency is a much bigger problem if what you're waiting for is life-saving information, and your biological clock is ticking because you don't have it.)

It's called the lethal lag time because people can die waiting. It behooves patients and their advocates to scour the web looking for new findings that haven't made it to us yet.

Even worse, once the information does hit the field, medical practice is very slow to evolve. The figure I've heard commonly quoted is that new practices take 17 years to become widely adopted.

So if you want to do everything in your power to maximize your odds, do not assume that every physician you talk to is fully up on everything. If you find something new, bring it to them and say, "I found this thing that we haven't discussed. What do you think?"

It looks like it won't be, but I learned a bunch about what the options would be.

I also had the whole-body bone scan, as planned, to check for any other possible "bone mets." Bottom line is that there were no big surprises. The sore spot on my arm is, as I suspected, a smaller bone met. This one's on the outside of the bone, not on the inside "eating out." So it's the kind that responds well to Interleuken, which I'm already expecting to get. So no additional treatment will be required.

There's also what they called a "tiny tiny" spot on my head; I don't know details but we've apparently caught it before it could have any influence on the overall picture.

Bottom line, the results of the bone scan very likely won't affect the overall plan. AND, ta-da, we've now scanned absolutely everything: all the organs and all the bones.

Today I completed the radiation treatments on the leg. And while at the hospital I've gotten pretty darn good at wheelchairing myself at a pretty good clip, which is by far the best exercise I've had recently – and I enjoy it.

I had a wonderful barbershop quartet practice tonight. I sure love to sing with my guys.

Re early mornings:

Both Monday and Tuesday I was 30 min. late for my 8 a.m. appointments.... I guess it's not easy to win against Boston morning traffic. So, for the Friday stress test, which is given once a day at 7:50 a.m., I'll stay overnight at a hotel. I'm REALLY glad I made THAT decision! I prefer not to have 3 of the 8 pre-surgery days begin with too little sleep and rush hour stress.

We also agreed it's time to replace the old mattress, because both of us are going to want comfort and restfulness. So we found a good price at a place that offers "no payments no interest" for a year.

p.s. The orthopedic surgeon was the high point of these days. She also has patients at Children's Hospital, so after we chatted a little she bent down and said, "Okay, now I'm going to check your pulse on your little feeties."

Thursday, March 1, 2007 12:13 AM

Tonight Ginny is at her favorite aunt's house ("Tante"), and tomorrow night I'll be away at the hotel near the hospital. So we have 2-1/2 days apart. That's healthy for both of us – helps us regroup and stay in touch with who we are.

Now, after 7 weeks of learning, diagnosis, scans and tests, the time has come. The prep is finished, and we're in the countdown of the last 6 nights before surgery.

And tonight I finally cried a bit.

Cried somewhat from fear: not terror, just a general knowing "Okay, we've done everything we can – what if it's not enough??" I acknowledged the feeling and let it go.

I cried somewhat out of emotion over all the incredible love my friends and family have shown me. I feel like I'm on a giant comforter of gentle support.

Most of all, I cried out of knowing that when I go under anesthesia, there's nothing more I can do, and that's scary. Dr. Wagner's team is going to remove that cancerous kidney, and I'll have nothing to say or do until I wake up.

And tonight after all that, near the end of the evening, I went to the tail end of my chorus's rehearsal. Lord, what a heartwarming experience that was. The sound of glorious harmony truly improved how I physically felt.

There must be some endorphin effect that arises when I hear really good close harmony – the kind where the chords ring with overtones. People said I looked noticeably better by the end of the rehearsal than 1/2 hour earlier.

Friend & author Lucy Jo Palladino PhD says crying for release is physically healthy. Says she saw a paper where onion tears were compared with emotional tears ("physic tears") and the emotional tears contained extra immune system stuff including T1 cells.

My googling didn't find a reference, but it matches my own experience: whenever I have a big cathartic release (for instance in a relationship breakthrough or in personal development courses I've taken from Landmark Education), completing something that's present or from the past, I always feel physically different, purged, cleansed, like a storm has ended and a new day is dawning.

Your love supports me in feeling strong and ready for it all. Bless you. Peace and love to you all, and thanks.

Friday, March 2, 2007 10:17 PM

BOZO OF THE MONTH AWARD – TWICE!

Prelude: Thursday dinner and pain

As planned, last night I stayed at the hotel. I had a WONDERFUL dinner there with Lindsey and her mom Sandy. It was great to spend time together, and they both gave me good advice about my swelling. It continues to be unreliable and at times debilitating. So not surprisingly, much of the conversation was about the leg. In my room, I could barely walk to the bathroom.

Which brings us to the Bozo of the Month Award: Femur heat – 2 bozo awards.

This is wonderful news. But it's the kind of wonderful news that makes me think MIT's gonna phone me and ask for their diploma back.

Award #1: When I woke up Thursday, this hit me.

My post-radiation instructions said not to heat the affected area, e.g. in a sauna or jacuzzi or a half-hour heating pad. I read it, I understood it, I strictly obeyed.

And then, every night, I slept all night on my nice snuggly HEATED MATTRESS PAD.

YA THINK THIS COULD HAVE SOMETHING TO DO WITH WHY MY MUSCLES HURT????

Say Ow, and confer the Bozo of the Month award. And read on.

Award #2: Today, between appointments, I was doing some computer work in the wheelchair, and I felt warmth on my thigh. Yes, boys and girls, I had the laptop in its usual position, on my thighs, with the maximum hot spot squarely placed on the sore end of my left thigh.

Confer the second Bozo OTM award.

I removed the computer immediately, and right now I'm typing atop a wooden board, atop a thick cushion.

So, folks, once again I have an answer to my recurring question

Laugh, Sing, and Eat Like a Pig

"What's going on here???" And once again the answer has nothing to do with kidney cancer.

Medical update 2: Appointments

Today I had the remaining qualification tests for the HDIL-2, which is now due to start in a few weeks (maybe March 26). These are tests designed to see whether my studly physique can handle the stress of the treatment. We'll get the answer soon.

Morning: I had the stress test. I will always remember this day as two visual images playing over and over and over: the Atlanta bus crash and Anna Nicole's casket being flown to the Bahamas. Why? Because a nuclear medicine "non-exercise stress test" is the most boring thing in the world: Do something, wait 20 minutes in the TV room, do something, wait 45 minutes in the TV room, lather, rinse, repeat. And over and over and over, those Breaking News items played on CNN Headline News.

I hardly remember the tests themselves ... it was the always exciting "now lie on your back for 20 minutes", interspersed with "Now we'll pump more of this into your IV."

Then I had my pulmonary function test. The scuba-like mouthpiece and lung capacity cylinder reminded me of a certain incident in April 1972, which is known to only a few people. :-)

Between appointments I also visited 12 Reisman, the floor where I'll spend 2 nights. Got to meet a couple of the nursing staff – always good to grease the wheels a little before doing business. The floor has a big poster/award about earning the prestigious 5 star award for customer satisfaction. (No, I don't know which award, but I like the sound of it.)

Here's hopin' I'll be completely over the leg thing by the end of the weekend! Surgery is now 3-1/2 days away.

Saturday, March 3, 2007 10:33 PM

My leg is doing DEFINITELY better, now that the secret heat sources have been removed. No more swollen muscles.

Dept of Transportation:

Behold the Hugo Rolling Walker. The "Hugoanywhere" Rolling Walker is a spectacular device. We bought one today at Costco, $96 instead of list price $155. For my current condition it works far better than a cane. The fold-up seat lets you stash a few portables in it, and the twin handles make it much easier than a cane: no wobbling! (And it has handbrakes, which are mainly useful to just lock it in place.) (It's not like I want to apply handbrakes while toodling around town.)

Of course it feels weird to be buying things I'd ordinarily expect to see in a nursing home, which is not a place I identify with. But I'm not committed to what I identify with – I'm committed to what works! And this thing does.

Dept of Transportation 2:

In wheelchairs, Kohl's gets a D – they have narrow chairs. At 220 lbs I'm not nearly a fatso, but I hardly fit into it.

- We discovered why the chairs are narrow: Kohl's aisles are, too. In the shirts & slacks section there was barely enough room to get through the rows.

- And there was no way to get a wheelchair into a dressing room, period.

- On the first chair we found, the front tire was off its rim. We took it to a checkout counter and talked with them, and left it with the wheel in the air so others would see and would not try to use it. When we left the store, it was back at the front door, still broken.

Sunday, March 4, 2007 8:45 PM

Surgery's Tuesday..... I must say I'm less full of brightness than I've been for the past few weeks. The surgery will be over in a blink, but that means the HDIL-2 is a few weeks away. And for that month-long treatment, I keep getting an image of being strapped into one of those rocket sleds that were used by X-15 test pilots: no matter how much you've prepared, once the test starts and the wind is blasting you in the face, you ride it out!

But now that I mention it, that's not an apt metaphor: if the HDIL is not going well, they just stop it immediately. Well, that's nice! I'm glad I spoke my concern, because then I saw it was bogus.

NPO day is here!

Good old "Nulla Per Os" – Latin for nothing by mouth. It's how the medicos have us enter surgery with a truly empty digestive system. Nothing but clear liquids, that is; and Jell-O counts as a liquid. So at wake-up Monday I get to take a marvelous system-clearing concoction. I'm to stick next to The Facilities most of the day, and have nothing to eat at all until surgery is past, approx 40 hrs. So I'll go from 6 weeks of "EAT EVERYTHING NOW!" to nuttin at all. Ought to be an interesting experience (not!)

I guess when they start surgery by inflating my teensy little belly with CO_2, they want no resistance AT ALL from gut contents. Fine with me – if the outcomes were better with painted toenails, I'd do that, too.

Rolling Walker, pt. 2:

This is a wondrous thing. Getting ready for the day, this morning, was completely different.

See, when you have a cane and a wobbly knee, you're left with about 1/2 a hand to carry anything with. With the walker I can load up a bunch of clothes, a coffee cup on the seat, etc., and move from room to room with both hands providing support on the walker's handles. Much less walking back and forth is required, and much less need for the bad leg to support the whole body's weight on each step.

Vaccine trial: As I mentioned in an early post, one treatment option is a new type of vaccine that's in the very early stages of research. Daughter Lindsey, who's working in an immunology lab at Mass General Hospital, asked what kind. I asked my oncologist, and he said it's a "dendritic cell/tumor fusion vaccine". (Oooooo-kay!) She responded "I wrote about that in my cancer immunology paper last year, too" and pasted in some text that was quite opaque to me but had a lovely rhythm. :-)

Monday, March 5, 2007 9:00 PM

Today I was beset by weasels nipping at my ankles, in almost every aspect of life. But now I'm in the hotel with Ginny and my mom, and it's time for a wonderful night of rest. And that's a good thing.

Ginny or Suede will be posting updates while I'm unable to. The hospital wing where I'll be staying is NOT in the wireless zone, so if there's no news until late in the day, don't have a cow. :-)

Chapter 3:
Facing Death – with Hope

Before the story continues I want to lay the emotional foundation. First I looked death squarely in the eye. Then, regardless of the odds, I chose hope.

◆   ◆   ◆

Facing Death

People who've faced imminent death share a certain awareness. If you've just joined those ranks, welcome. You should know, some of us live through it, and some don't. You will be one or the other.

In my most desperate moments one question gripped my mind: "What can be said that will make any difference?"

I vividly recall realizing it was over. In my speeches I talk about realizing I'd never see my daughter's children, and they'd never know me. I talk about lying awake that January night, realizing my memorial service might be a few months away. Would it be May? September? What would the weather be like that day, as people gathered?

My father's memorial service was fresh in my mind, so my thoughts were vivid. What would my mom's face look like as she said goodbye to her son?

"Prepare yourself to follow me."

I'd had some preparation for this moment.

In my 40s for some reason I took an interest in aging and death. In the library I'd found recordings of Harvard psychologist Richard Alpert, an associate of Timothy Leary; Alpert went to Tibet, found a guru, and took the Sanskrit name Ram Dass, "servant of God." In "Approaching Death" he cited a tombstone inscribed,

As I am now,
so you will be.
Prepare yourself
to follow me.

He talked about ministering to many people as they went through this final transition during the AIDS epidemic, and more years working in hospice. Somehow his words rang with wisdom for me as he combined the perspectives of Harvard, ancient Egyptian scriptures, and modern practices of Tibetan monks, often expressing them with the humor of a New England Jew.

My sister Suede was a similar influence closer to home. Like Ram Dass she had worked with AIDS patients during their final passages. (Her first album includes the deeply moving song "The Ones Who Aren't Here," which was written during the AIDS epidemic.) "Everyone deals with this differently," she said. "There's no right way."

When I realized I was in that state their words came to mind. "Death soon" was so real that I asked my doctor what it would feel like at the end. He thought I meant pain, so he assured me I'd be kept comfortable. I said no, I was thinking about the passage itself: "What will it be like at the end? Will my lungs shut down so I'll be short of breath? Something else?"

Radical acceptance

I was prepared to let my experience be my experience, expecting nothing, with nothing wrong: my feelings would be whatever they were, and I would stay mindful.

Terry Wilson, a member of my ACOR kidney cancer group, told me of "radical acceptance," a concept discussed by Dr. Marsha Linehan. It combines western cognitive-behavioral techniques (altering how we look at things) with eastern practices for mindfulness, distress tolerance and acceptance. Radical means complete and absolute. And that's the space I found myself in: "All right, this is what's so. Let's get to work."

Acceptance of one's situation, seeing it as it is, doesn't mean giving up. To the contrary, it gives one a firm place to stand, attached to reality, with no energy-sapping resistance. Here's the point of view I came to.

- **Am I dying? Yes.** Ram Dass quotes someone who said "Being born is like setting sail on a ship whose purpose is to go out in the ocean and sink."

- **Am I dying *now*, of this cancer?** Nobody knows. You can learn about the odds, more or less, but odds apply to large populations, not individuals.

- **I won't die of cancer if I live long enough for something else to get me.** My ACOR patient community quickly taught me that the game is to live long enough for something else to get you. This might seem crazy, but think about it: if you feel trapped, like you can't escape cancer, it helps to know it might not get you. Examples:

  - If you live long enough to be killed by a bus, cancer didn't kill you. HA!

  - If you live long enough for a cure to be developed, the cancer didn't kill you.

  - You might live long enough for a treatment that makes it a chronic condition, not fatal. (Yes, there are some cancers that are now managed as chronic diseases – they're not fatal!)

  - It's not unusual for an autopsy to discover a cancer that nobody knew was there. They died of something else. Cancer doesn't always kill people.

- **I had some warning. Some people don't.** 1200 people woke up today in the US and got dressed, not realizing it was for the last time: by midnight they'll fall to sudden cardiac death. They had no chance to think things out, prepare, respond. I, at least, had a warning, a chance to get it in gear.

- **You might get better for no apparent reason.** It happens. A small percentage of all cancers disappear spontaneously, and science doesn't know why. *It is not scientific to say there's no*

> ## "Talk honestly about how you feel every day"
>
> Reflecting on these days later, my wife Ginny had these thoughts.
>
> We could see that the cancer had spread. We were both sort of silent, in our own worlds, thinking about the possibility of him not being there. We had a few nights of crying.
>
> You have to talk honestly about how you feel every day. We're sort of silly people anyway, so it wasn't a stretch to continue to be that way. He loves to do plays on words. It wasn't hard for me to fall into that pattern. We all die someday. We want to have the best time we can while we're here.
>
> We thought, well, if there are only 6 weeks or 18 weeks, let's live it. We checked the wills, the power of attorney. Dave took on the fight. I would support him any I way I could.

chance of this. (I wouldn't bet my house on it, but my mind was completely open to the possibility.)

• **Until I die, I'm alive every day.** That's certain.

"I don't know. But we will try."

At a Christmas party in 2008 I met a kidney cancer specialist from another hospital, a marvelous grandfatherly Greek. We talked about hope, and he said he's changed his answer when patients ask if they'll get better.

He used to say it's not likely, and he'd watch the life go out of them. "Now I tell them, 'I don't know. But we will *try*. Will you work with me?'"

And he adds, "Just one thing: if we succeed, you must *drive carefully*. We don't want to save you and have it wasted!"

You don't have to survive, you know. You may decide you've had enough, now is your time, and you choose to let go.

Or, you can choose to try everything. Or try until you've had enough. To me the question is, do you have something worth living for? A future worth living to see? If so, let's get to work.

◆　◆　◆

Laugh, Sing, and Eat Like a Pig

About Hope

Hope is a resource. A real, scientifically verified resource.

Jerome Groopman MD's excellent book *The Anatomy of Hope* cites evidence from well controlled experiments: when challenged, patients' bodies perform differently based on their minds' expectation.

We're not just talking about their experience of pain – scientists measured substantial difference in their **physiological response**, comparable in strength to a drug. Dr. Groopman calls hope "a catalyst in the crucible of cure" and concludes, **"There is an authentic biology of hope."**

Movingly, he describes decades of being with patients as they faced probable death, and his journey as a physician learning to help them deal with it. Today he writes:

> Hope, unlike optimism, is rooted in **unalloyed reality. ...**
> Hope acknowledges the significant obstacles and deep
> pitfalls along the path. True hope has no room for delusion.

> Clear-eyed, hope gives us the courage to confront our
> circumstances and the capacity to sumount them. For all
> my patients, **hope, true hope, has proved as important as
> any medication.**

I'll repeat: hope is now science, not speculation. If you don't believe it, read the book.

He says hope has two components – belief and expectation. I'll paraphrase it: when you believe there's no hope, your biology shifts: it's as if your cells give up, your system gives up; your body doesn't do as well as it could **if it had hope.**

Being Scientific About the Unknown

Science can get arrogant, saying "If we don't have evidence for something, don't believe it." But there's another saying: "Absence of evidence is not evidence of absence." History is full of things that were true long before science figured it out. Consider:

- Oxygen was oxygen, doing what it does, long before Priestley figured it out in 1774.

- Bacteria were bacteria, doing what they do, long before scientists proposed the germ theory of medicine in the 1800s. (When bacteria were proposed, science was incredulous: infections were being caused by an invisible evil creature? Why, that's witchcraft! But it was real. Science just hadn't figured it out yet.)

- DNA was DNA, doing what it does, long before Watson and Crick figured it out in the 1950s.

And hope was doing what it does – whatever that is – before the experiments Groopman cites. Perhaps it's related to how PNI (psychoneuroimmunology) works: thoughts (psych) measurably affect the nervous system, which measurably affects the immune system.

Reality Is What It Is – Whether We Know It or Not

This is the first instance in this book of a recurring theme:

Reality is what it is,
regardless of what we think
and whether we know it or not.

There may be pathways to recovery that science hasn't found yet. And one of them might have your name on it. Or not: how would I know? The point is that there's a world of undiscovered reality, and not a soul can tell you something won't happen. They can tell you it's bloody unlikely, but they can't say never.

Besides, what are you going to do when science runs out of answers? That's the world I live in. My oncologist, Dr. David McDermott, told me my odds of a relapse were 50%, and we have no way to predict the outcome.

I went home and thought … and I wrote a post about evidence-based medicine. It began:

> "On the fringes of medical knowledge, lives are at stake
> and medicine doesn't have the answers yet. What do
> you do?"

"We Came to Give You Hope"

My best friend is a rigorous and deep-thinking scientist named Dorron Levy. He's a former co-worker, a brilliant guy who now lives in Israel. When he learned of my diagnosis he shared my PatientSite login with his brother, a leading physician in Israel, who read my data and told him I was basically screwed.

Dorron's family was shaken, and as described in the last chapter, they visited for a long weekend. It was costly: four short-notice plane tickets, hotel and all. And since at the time I still had the financial stress of owning two houses (I had just moved back to the Boston area from Minnesota), they insisted on buying all our meals.

I recently said to him "You must have felt you were coming to say goodbye." He replied, "Nothing could be farther from the truth. I was certain you would make it. We came to give you hope."

Hearing this from a high priest of evidence made my jaw drop. He said, "Dave, in physics right now there are two contending factions – reductionism and emergence. Reductionists want to eliminate all confounding variables to get repeatable results. Emergence is the study of what tiny influences lead to new patterns as the chaos unfolds." His action in "giving hope" was an injection into the chaos.

"An incredible life force"

In 2009 my oncologist, Dr. McDermott – one of the best scientists in the world for this disease – capped it off, saying "You have an incredible life force that everyone who worked on your case was aware of."

Amazed, I thought to myself, "Where's the evidence for *that*?" But his word's good enough for me. Until you decide it's your time to go, don't give up hope. You have no idea what might happen.

♦   ♦   ♦

And so, we began treatment. First, remove the diseased kidney.

Chapter 4: Surgery

March 6 – April 2, 2007

Tuesday, March 6, 2007, 12:20 PM

Hi all, Ginny here.

Suede, Anne (Mom) and I are at the hospital while Dave is happily snoozing away. He told me he was going to be giggling during surgery. He was relaxed and happy while waiting for the doctors. He is at Beth Israel hospital in Boston in the Feldberg/Reisman building. His room # is not known to us at this time, but will let everyone know when we get it. He is expected to go home Thursday or Friday. Dave is sooo grateful for all the warm thoughts and wishes sent his way. Actually we all feel your loving support. Thank you from all of us. Ginny

Tuesday, March 6, 2007 3:40 PM

And a 3:45pm PS from sister Suede – the mighty trio awaits word from the O.R. which we imagine will be coming soon. Of course we'll pass that along immediately. As Ginny said, Dave's spirits were great as he waited to go in. Also, as Ginny said we're all so grateful for your concern, love, support and great posts in the guest book. They mean so much to us all, especially Dave! What a team we are! More as we get it – promise.

Tuesday, March 6, 2007 3:59 PM

We JUST met with Dave's surgeon, Dr. Wagner, who let us know that all went well. Dave is in recovery for the next two hours. We'll see him as soon as we can and keep you posted here.

Again, all went well!

Suede, Ginny and Mom

Wednesday, March 7, 2007 1:29 AM

Warmest greetings to the Team!

Suede here...

Now that Ginny, Mom, Lindsey and beau Jon and I have had some time with Dave post-op I wanted to share some more details while Dave is hopefully resting peacefully after a long day. Knowing Dave has been so honest and complete in his sharing with us all I am certain he'd want me to do so as well.

We arrived at the hospital this morning at 8:45 to get Dave checked in. He was in surgery from about 10:30am until 4pm – approximately 5.5 hours. The procedure took longer than expected for two reasons: 1) the adrenal gland was involved with the tumor and was also removed (as planned) making for two surgeries in one for all intents and purposes; and, 2) the tumor had attached to the wall of the bowel as well as the psoas muscle which embraces the side of the lumbar spine and had to be very carefully peeled away from both surfaces. Dr. Wagner was concerned that he might have to effectively start all over with a more commonly used incision but was remarkably able to perform the very intricate procedure laparoscopically. This man is a wonder. Dave is in excellent hands, indeed. All went very well, albeit more involved and longer than originally expected.

Dave was in recovery for over two hours and we finally got to see him at about 7pm. He was in a great deal of pain which is to be expected after such an intense procedure. The hospital team worked relentlessly to make him comfortable. In fact, the first step out of surgery is pain management and we are hopeful and confident that he will feel much better tomorrow and even better the day after that.

I am pleased to report that Dave's sense of humor was very present, as usual. As he was wheeled into his room and saw Mom there he said "Mommy, they HURT me!" and then was scheming on how to punch the Dr. as Dr. Wagner wisely moved Dave's cane out of his reach.

Dave is due to be up and out of bed tomorrow. Ginny is at Dave's side tonight, sleeping right in the room with him. He will be in the hospital Wednesday and Thursday (likely) and be on his way home Friday if Dr. Wagner feels he is strong enough to be released.

We put several of your cards up in his room already and more will go up tomorrow. Dave is surrounded by your love and that has made a huge difference for him and for all of us.

I hope I have covered everything. Feel free to post any questions here and I'll do my best to answer them.

More to come, my friends.

Much love to you all,

Suede

Wednesday, March 7, 2007 9:17 AM

GOOOOOOOD MORNING, BOSTON!!!!!!!!!!!!

Laparoscopic kidney surgery: amazing

Dr. Drew Wagner is the surgeon who did the deed for me. He does the really fancy stuff, laparoscopic kidney removal. Three little incisions to stick the instruments through, and a 2-3" bikini incision (yes, I have a bikini scar, and no you can't see it) through which they remove the culprit.

Now, here's the thing, and I really want you to get this: they inflate the belly to give themselves room, then they stick the tools in through the tiny incisions, and do the work by watching it on a TV. They remove the organ (which is large) by basically snipping it off, putting it in a Baggie, zipping it up, and sliding it out through the bikini cut.

Of course, they have to do this with surgical precision, in the dark except for the flashlight they stuck in there. And here's another thing: the TV is 2D, but your guts (including the location of blood vessels etc) are 3D. And p.s., you don't get to accidentally bump into anything with your knife.

I had a unique opportunity to experience what laparoscopy is like. Beth Israel Deaconess has an amazing simulation and training center, where students can actually handle laparoscopic equipment. The very first training exercise involves holding two long-armed gripper tools, and all you have to do is use them to pick up some little white beans and put them in a cup. A foot away, and several inches higher.

And the rest of your crazy old world out there.

I'll keep this brief – lots more details in the coming days. I just want to say that last night I was in BAD pain, and today I'm not. I feel terrific. (Of course, it helps that I'm on morphine.)

I hear tell that I was a complicated case, which took 6 hrs, not the 3-1/2 typical. When I got to my room and saw Mom, I said (in my creaky, hoarse voice), "Mommie they hurt me!!!"

Ginny stayed in the room with me overnight, on a recliner chair, playing a CD of wonderful Reiki music. It did me a world of good to reach over and touch her, or for her to crack one of her giggle-maker jokes.

Today they're taking me off the morphine, and I'll start actually SWALLOWING (not just sipping), and I'll start on toast and crackers (wow, solids!).

More later. Thanks to EVERY SINGLE ONE OF YOU for your support. It looks like we made good use of every bit of support.

That's plenty rough when you can see what you're doing. But when you're good at it, they put a drape over the plastic box that contains all this, and you lose all depth perception because now you're watching it on TV.

Then, don't get nervous or anything, but just remember that while you're trying to do this, the patient is bleeding (or might be) and every extra minute under anesthesia adds risk. So don't screw up. Oh, and pick up that bean you just dropped, because it rolled under the pancreas and it's really a piece of tumor. Or something.

And then they tell you that this is the first of the laparoscopic training hurdles. You don't get to move to the next machine until you can move 10 beans from lower left to the cup in one minute, with no depth perception.

Until I tried this myself, it had never dawned on me that a surgeon has to be damned athletic as well as smart. And when I think of this guy going into my inflated belly through these little incisions and delicately peeling that super-aggressive tumor off the bowel, and off that muscle attached to my spine.... both of which the tumor was on the verge of invading... and then the adrenal gland got away, and had to be chased down ... well, the surgery took 5.5 hours, almost had to convert to the rib-removing version, and yet I went home two days later.

Is this guy good, or what?

Wednesday, March 7, 2007 10:01 PM

LONG CRANKY DAY

Sorry for the delay on this. Had a number of delays that, well, delayed us. :-)

Good news of progression today, and visits from some fun nearbys. By the time it was over I was frustrated (not ENOUGH happened today) but I'm again ready for a good night's sleep.

Medically, I got weaned from the morphine, and was moved (midday) to Percocet. Percocet isn't as strong so I'm ouchy, but MUCH better than a few days ago.

Everyone I saw today said "You look GREAT" or "You're a new man!" And indeed, I felt like one!

Because I don't have wireless in this hospital room, I've typed these notes on a computer and Ginny carries it to a wireless lobby to post it on CaringBridge.

HOMECOMING THURSDAY??

We're still hoping that my doc will release me tomorrow! It'd be great to be back home.

Thursday, March 8, 2007 12:03 PM

Hi, y'all - a quick update from moi. (This building doesn't have wireless, but if you go to the sunroom at the magic corner, you can get wireless from the building next door.)

It's likely that I'll be going home today. Had a very rough night due to miscommunication problems, which led to my not getting the right dose of meds. Now it's fixed. I'm up and walking about on the floor.

Thursday, March 8, 2007 7:55 PM

People, let me tell you, I am TIRED. We came home tonight and I got a go-home boost to my narcotic prescription, and no I'm not the least bit intrigued by the opportunity to be playful with this aspect of things; I just want to feel rested and restored again, and without pain.

Frankly, y'all, I'm too pooped to do a thing tonight. See ya this weekend, in the wires. Thank you so much for all your cards & guestbook posts that come in.

Mom and Ginny have been powerhouses of dedicated support. I'm blessed.

p.s. The leg pain is 98% gone, btw. Pretty amazing.

Silos, Caring, and Coordination

An often-cited problem with healthcare today is "silos" – the idea that medicine is so specialized that people in one department may know practically nothing about the patient except their own specialty. If you're ever hospitalized, you'd better be aware of this and be vigilant, until you satisfy yourself that your hospital doesn't have the problem.

In an interview for this book, Dr. Sands put it this way: "As Dave was struggling with his therapy and his leg fracture, he expressed frustration about our healthcare system. 'Why doesn't Dr X know Y about me? Who's coordinating all this?' To some extent, the primary care physician should do this. But patients with complex cases may need someone else to act as a case manager."

And that's at one of America's best hospitals, with staff who truly care. So imagine what it's like at lesser places.

In my case, some of the staff on my post-surgical floor had no idea that my leg was in the process of breaking – one nurse asked me to stand up, without fetching my walker. (Nobody'd told her, and she hadn't read my chart.) Another knew I'd had surgery but didn't know about the cancer. At another time I was prescribed a medication I wasn't supposed to get, because of the treatments I was getting.

A common cause of this in America today is that there's no insurance billing code for care coordination, because billing codes are based on diagnoses, not treatments. In my view that's disgusting, but there you have it. Be aware; don't assume somebody is on top of everything – even if they're sharp people. Believe me, the business of healthcare is not necessarily oriented around patients' needs – not even legitimate medical needs.

Sunday, March 11, 2007 4:25 PM

Hi folks – can't believe it's been 3 days, and I haven't posted anything since I got home! I guess the signs are clear: I've been really tired, moving slowly, learning day by day to manage what hurts and what doesn't.

One thing's become clear: there are two different questions about well-being. There's "Is the patient's medical and physical recovery on track?" Separate from that, there's "How's the patient doing? How does he say he's doing, how is his wife doing, how's his family doing? Are they on track to recovery, or worried, or what?"

Sunday, March 11, 2007 10:08 PM

Now (March 11), 5 days post surgery, the surgeon is happy. He says generally things are progressing as they should. But that skips a LOT of details. It'll take a few days.

Tomorrow I'll post on what's happened since I got home. Upcoming chapters:

GETTING THROUGH THE DAY

- The Hugo Rolling Walker
- The splint pillow
- A cough preventer

GETTING AROUND THE HOUSE

- Using the cane vs the Rolling Walker
- Bathroom at night

GETTING THROUGH THE NIGHT
The Pee Journal (This is the key to the whole thing.)

- Getting out of bed many times a night
- Sitting up when you have incision pain
- Using a wood block for support

- Shortening the path from bedside to john

- Why does it happen so often??

— Dave

p.s. I gotta tell you, every day at home there have been days when "How's it going??" has been very up-and-down. Do something that hurts, at the wrong moment, and your plans for the rest of the day can be tanked. Or something suddenly is NOT hurting, and a world opens up.

Thursday, March 15, 2007

Medical quick summary:

- Kidney removal surgery process is just about complete. I got 5 stars for having my recovery go perfectly: off meds ahead of schedule, etc. BUT, I got a little chest cold, and MAN do the incisions hurt if you cough the wrong way.

- It's been wonderful having Mom here since March 5. She leaves Sat. 3/17.

- I won't go into details of the past week, but it's true that in a recovery, it's a BIG DEAL to manage the return of one's normal digestive functions.

- #1 medical issue of the moment is the left knee, which has been unstable. Lots to learn there about self-awareness and how to walk consciously. I'll probably have an orthopedic consult next week.

- Next item is continued prep for HDIL-2 (High-Dosage Interleukin 2). We see the oncology team Monday 4pm.

- 2pm that same day, I'm getting an echocardiogram (ultrasound of the heart) to clarify something from the stress test I had before surgery.

11:23 AM: Non-medical

Last night I'd felt like not visiting my chorus practice (they're heading off to competition this weekend) but Mom and Ginny convinced me, and I'm glad I went. It was so energizing and uplifting!

Sunday, March 18, 2007 9:58 PM

What a week, what a weekend, what a day.

My mom left yesterday, after 12 days. She is one of these amazing women who causes a room to become neat and organized by simply standing in it. And, she is my mother, and this is the first time I've ever had her to myself for 12 days, since I was 2 years old. It was wonderful.

Kidney surgery is complete and resolved. As of Friday I can roll over in bed. I have no discomfort that would keep me from doing anything.

My left knee is still a big interference in life. I can't walk without cane or walker, and in any case I can't walk any distance to speak of. So this becomes a show-stopper re returning to work, or going to a store, or anything else driving-related, by myself.

Every afternoon I've had one or two naps – I didn't have much get-up-n-go. But day after day unexpected new recovery signs would show up. (A good example is being able to roll over in bed, where a week earlier I needed special methods to get in or out of bed.)

Somehow, out of nowhere, I woke up today feeling like it's time to re-engage the outside world. I want to start taking short little drives again, to confirm that I have the belly strength to move from pedal to pedal. I want to start re-engaging with work, in whatever chunks are workable.

Today was pretty much on the move, all day. Played late in bed, got up and did several things at home, showered & dressed, picked up a prescription, went to Olive Garden and headed over to Costco and did a fair amount of damage (mostly groceries), including a $39 (!!!) DVD player for the living room TV. (Costco has THE BEST shopping scooters.) Brought the goods home, and spent over an hour on the floor wrestling with cables and remotes, getting the new toy to play nicely with the old toys.

(I can hear my mom right now saying, with alarm, "JEEZE, Dave!" Don't worry, mom; as with everything I did last week, it only went as far as I felt comfortable.)

So here it is, 10pm Sunday, about to post this, then hit the hay.

Tomorrow (Monday) we have Dr appointments for

- orthopedic surgeon to re-assess the knee
- getting an echocardiogram to confirm my status to go into the HDIL treatments, whenever that happens.
- oncology team, to re-assess my whole status

I'd love to see things continue on this trend.... but we shall see what we see. It's a day-by-day game.

Tuesday, March 20, 2007 12:43 PM

Summary of Monday's appointments at the hospital

The surgery recovery is almost perfect.

My cardiology / stress test results are fine. In fact, they said they WERE going to start me on HDIL next Monday!

But last week I pointed out my ongoing leg trouble, so yesterday they took new x-rays, and it looks like the femur bone met might be growing (or not – they can't tell from the x-ray).

There has definitely been more bone loss near the knee, but that can be caused by the radiation treatment. Regardless, we need to protect the bone: keep as much weight off it as possible, to prevent fracture.

A physical therapist is coming to visit tomorrow, to train me on walker / wheelchair / crutch methods.

The forearm swelling (another bone met) has increased noticeably – we knew THAT much without a doctor.

So before we move ahead with HDIL, they want to know: do I

suddenly have some fast-growing tumor spots? If so, they want to stop those before doing the HDIL.

So, tomorrow we're getting another whole-torso scan, to compare with the previous one. We'll see the doc next Monday to see what's next.

If the scan says "no rapid growth" I start Interleukin two weeks from now! (April 2)

If not, we start another treatment that has strong short-term benefits, which will last long enough to cover the HDIL treatment. And we see how that goes.

♦   ♦   ♦

Psych / mental update

I'm finally getting annoyed with all this – REALLY annoyed. I know this is a stage people naturally go through. I'm just getting sick and tired of beating one thing and, every single stinkin time, having something else come up out of nowhere. NOT FAIR! Angry! Ticked off! Disgusted! etc.

And, I know that resisting things will do no good. So I'm looking at accepting that that's how my cancer is going, while at the same time being angry about it.

As with everything that's come before, I'll learn what there is to learn and use every resource I have (including all you) to beat it.

♦   ♦   ♦

A quote in a book sent by Guestbooker Leslie Harkins (*There's No Place Like Hope*):

> I know God won't give me anything I can't handle.
> I just wish He didn't trust me so much.
>
> – Mother Teresa

Sunday, March 25, 2007 10:18 PM

Monday (tomorrow) we get the news about whether I have new

aggressive tumor growths that will keep me from starting the high-dose Interleukin-2 on April 2.

New growth is suspected because my femur wall is now paper thin (subject to fracture soon), and my left arm is increasingly ouchy and sensitive to the slightest touch.

Last week's CAT scan checked the whole torso for changes in the lung metastases or any new mets elsewhere.

What the heck is goin' on here? This is supposed to be KIDNEY cancer, not Miscellaneous-Other-Places cancer. Evasive little bastard.

OKAY, MOOD CHECK:

I hereby declare that I strongly object to the following:

- pain, whether steady or intermittent

- being unable to walk unassisted

- the growing inventory of rehab equipment in this house: cane, rolling walker, full-bore wheelchair, and a weird but useful thing called a Platform Walker .... especially since all that is caused by the leg problem, NOT the blasted kidney.

- the incessant cycle of mastering one state of affairs and then almost immediately being hit with a new issue.

- increasing inability to know what the near future holds.

But as I've said before, I also know it doesn't do any good to resist that something is so. What gives us the most power is to grant that it's so, even while granting our own feelings about it, too.

I must say, it does make a notable difference whenever someone from my life reaches out and asks how I'm doing. Thank you, very much, no kidding, really. When I face a moment of uncertainty it helps to know y'all are out there!

Honestly, I never knew I had so many friends who remembered me and gave a rat's patoot. Your visits and notes move me.

Monday, March 26, 2007 10:09 PM

I'M A GO FOR HDIL-2 STARTING MONDAY

Reviewing last week's CT scan, the team says I do have new tumor growth happening in the metastases in my lungs. That's consistent with the noticeable growth also seen in my bone mets. In other words, the cancer is now on the move:

- My smallest lung lesion (1/3″) has grown to 2/3″

- The largest lesion has grown (but nowhere near doubling in radius).

- There are no new tumor sites (which is good)

The team's conclusion is that the best thing is still to admit me Monday and proceed with the HDIL-2 – but keep an extra-close eye out for any indications of my tumor growth continuing.

If (perhaps after the first week) they find the growth is continuing, and there's no sign that the tumors are responding to the Interleukin, then

- stop the HDIL

- send me home

- start me on one of the more conventional therapies (Sutent, in pill form) which has the best chance of stopping the new growth immediately.

I get a very strong feeling that my oncology team (two superb doctors and a beyond-superb research coordinator nurse) knows my case (including my personality) in great detail, and is deeply committed to me and a successful outcome, and having it work the way I want. How great is that?

Mood Check 1: Extremely anxious

Despite what I've said for months about wanting HDIL, now that I'm facing actually throwing myself into the HDIL maelstrom, I found myself not just scared but really grumpy and anxious. HDIL is not a nice thing to anticipate, and there's no better option

54

available. In some ways it's like being told that it's time to walk the plank because the plank is the best they can offer me.

Mood Check 2: Settled and calm

In that state of mind, I was mildly obnoxious and jerky to my wife and everyone around me for a couple of hours. I realized: In this moment I'm severely confronted by the reality that although HDIL has the best odds, I'm still wrapped up in those fears.

But, as mega-nurse Kendra said, "It's bad, but it's a short bad – it's over in a week, then you have one more week, and that's the end of it."

And I knew all that two months ago. I'm just confronted by the fact that it's Now.

In this space, what was there for me was a more sober awareness that this is it, really. It's happening, just as I expected, except it's quite real.

I consciously let go of being in control. I already have all the information there is, and now it's time to jump off that cliff.

Evening: I venture forth for dinner, in a wheelchair

For the first time today, we put the wheelchair in the car. For no good reason at all I have a revulsion at being "a guy in a wheelchair" (it makes no sense; I never claimed to be sensible). But on the way home we stopped for supper, and I was surprised that it all went very well.

So what works, generally, is to NOT trust my senseless expectations (they're nuts) and just stay in touch with what I want (what I'm committed to).

After high school, a summer girlfriend hand-wrote me a wonderful booklet of aphorisms, Summer Revelations. One of them was perfect for this moment:

> "If you must doubt, doubt your doubts –
> never your beliefs."

Laugh, Sing, and Eat Like a Pig

Wednesday, March 28, 2007 10:15 AM

Today's a pretty vigorous day. Yesterday was the opposite. So it goes: one day at a time. My concerns about entering treatment are gone. Funny.... I realized I had this mental image that next Monday was some sort of impenetrable wall, where I go into treatment and beyond that it's all unknowable. But now I know I'm going in on 4/2, and coming home Sunday 4/8 (Easter) or earlier. When I think of so many people who've undergone years and years of treatment, some much worse than mine, it puts a new perspective on it.

And, not everyone has the side effects... I've been living as if they're certain, but they're not.

◆   ◆   ◆

A friend forwarded me the story of a man in Canada that has remarkable similarities to mine. He ended up having to have a leg amputation because of damage from a kidney cancer met, but he survived. Holy cow, if he can beat it ... my challenges seem a wee bit less challenging! And another friend tells of someone with cancer – when someone asks "How are you doing?" he responds "I'm fine except for this TEMPORARY cancer!"

Wednesday, March 28, 2007 10:17 PM

Yes, two posts in one day.

One day at a time, right? After being wiped out all day Tuesday, today I was up 'n' at 'em continuously from 7 a.m. to 10 p.m., with one 90 min nap after lunch. This is the first time that's happened since my decline started.

And, I GOT TO DRIVE! Twice.

I needed a haircut before going into the month-long treatment, and Ginny said "Would you like to drive?" She figured out how to get the wheelchair (and me) into the car, and we did it.

Then, bolder than ever, during supper I called a chorus friend and asked if he'd meet me at our rehearsal place and help me get the chair out of the car, so I could attend and listen. He said yes,

56

so I got to listen to chorus rehearsal AND let Ginny stay at home and rest for a couple of much-needed hours.

But I figure, I might as well start now making the Big Recovery.... no reason to wait until the hospitalization actually starts!

Friday, March 30, 2007 5:44 PM

OKAY, *CHILL!* THIS IS JUST HOW IT GOES! Now I've REALLY had enough of this.

I know, I gotta get over that, because as I've been saying for months, this is just how it goes. We get news, we incorporate it into our knowledge, we see whether the plan needs to change, and we move forward, continuing to do what we can.

This note isn't the best news, but it doesn't change the treatment plan: Last night I learned that I have some mets that we hadn't yet known about. Recently I said last week's CAT scan showed no new tumor sites. Today I learned that was correct, but only in the areas that had been scanned before. Two other mets exist in areas that hadn't been scanned before. The first showed up just outside the pelvis. (This is the first time the pelvis has been imaged.) The scan showed part of my thigh, including a met in the right thigh. (It doesn't hurt – it's just there.) At the other end (my head), there's another tiny bony met, on the skull. Wouldn't that news annoy you? Pisses me off. But that's what's so, whether I like it or not. So we include it in what's so and refocus on the goal of "N.E.D." (no evidence of disease) and move forward.

◆　　◆　　◆

Meanwhile, here I sit, doing better than ever: This is my third day straight of having good energy all day, and being productive (relatively) and focused (as much as I ever am. :-) I'm better than ever at getting around the house in my chair and platform walker, and (best of all) today the wheelchair company delivered a part they overlooked: a big gel cushion to coddle my tender butt.

I also got the Minnesota house listed for rent again (current lease expires 4/30), and set up a short-term "for sale" listing in case a buyer pops up before a renter does.

I'm glad I'm ready to go in for treatment now, not later! There's that lucky shoulder x-ray again, way back in January. I'm so glad to be several weeks farther along in the treatment schedule.

Saturday, March 31, 2007

Beautiful day today. After staying in bed with Ginny as late as we felt like, I went to part of a coaching session with my barbershop chorus. At break time they sang to me: "You'll never walk alone." It was moving.

I sang much of the afternoon. My breathing was good.

♦   ♦   ♦

Major mental discovery today: Way back when, I cited all the things I've read about HDIL that said the "side effects are often severe." I just realized that it says OFTEN, not USUALLY "are severe."

In other words, they really truly might not be severe. (They might, but they really might not be.)

Once again, it's a good thing I don't take my thoughts and concerns too seriously. Reality is reality, whether or not I know it, and regardless of what I think.

♦   ♦   ♦

One reason I like my oncologist:

Yesterday for the umpteenth time I sent him an email with more questions. Mind you, this is a busy guy with many patients like me and hundreds of other responsibilities. The following email exchange ensued:

> McDermott: "RCC [my type of kidney cancer] does not typically spread to muscle, but aggressive RCC can."

> Me: "Thank you. I'm acutely aware that I can be a lot to handle. I respect your time and skill and judgment. It's just that I ain't never done this before. :)"

> Him: "No problem. I am glad to field your questions."

58

Monday, April 2, 2007 6:43 AM

We're on the way!

◆　　◆　　◆

I didn't note it in CaringBridge at the time, but something disturbing happened in the middle of this month. Here's what I added – but not until September 25:

Shortly before we went in for IL-2, a strange growth appeared in the middle of my tongue. At first I thought it was one of those thick-lump cold sores, but this one didn't go away. And then a few days before we went to the hospital (literally less than a week), it seemed to swell, becoming a lump the size of a pea.

Carefully prodding with a popsicle stick (or something), Ginny and I discovered that it was actually mushroom-shaped, with a smaller round stem emerging from the tongue, and a "cap" growing off of that stem. Not your typical cold sore.

We showed it to the docs when we went in to the hospital, and asked about taking a biopsy. They said "Let's see how the IL-2 goes first."

And during that first week of IL-2, it shrank, receded, and disappeared.

We'll never know what it was, but I strongly suspect it was a metastasis, growing out of my tongue muscle.

Remember that it's rare for mets to grow in muscle – that only happens in the most aggressive cancers. I later found out that I had a 1" met in my right thigh muscle, so it's entirely feasible that I might have ended up with a 1" met growing out of my tongue muscle.

I literally shudder to think what might have happened if I hadn't been ready for IL-2 when that thing emerged. Would I like to have that mushroom thing growing out of my tongue for 6 weeks? I don't think so.

Chapter 5: Participating in My Care Online

Healthcare may be the least "online" industry we have, and I have a sneaking suspicion that's related to why our costs keep going up.

Throughout the first phase of this adventure, I made extensive use of PatientSite, my hospital's "patient portal." Portal is the industry term for a website that lets someone view a bunch of stuff, and "patient portal" is how a patient views a bunch of patient stuff. PatientSite is mine, and my primary physician Danny Sands was one of its creators long ago.

Discussing it for this book, Dr. Sands said, "Patients use our system mainly to get test results, but it also provides them with problem lists, medication lists, and so on. It went live in April 2000, and our system has been operating longer than any other institution's. Various others are now doing similar things, especially Cleveland, Kaiser, and Geisinger."

"Long ago" is apt, because it was designed around the turn of the century, and hasn't been upgraded much since then: it's hard to find any other website that looks so "1999." BUT, it's a heck of a lot more than most hospitals offer in 2010, and all I knew at the time was that it gave me a much-needed opportunity to be involved, to be engaged, to have some sense of participating in what the doctors could see. I implore every hospital to get it in gear and offer patients and families visibility into the medical record – and I urge patients and families to demand it.

Here are excerpts of two CaringBridge posts that mentioned it. The first bears repeating from Chapter 2.

February 6, 2007

As many of you know, my hospital (Beth Israel Deaconess) has a wonderful secure patient website www.PatientSite.org where parts of my medical records are visible to me, including CAT scan and MRI reports, and I can send and receive secure emails with the physicians. It's an incredibly open process, which really relieves me of wondering "what they know that I don't know."

> "Patients with access to their own medical records, test results, and documentation are more empowered to help their providers as well as themselves and are a critical part of the team."
>
> — Kendra Bradley, Research Coordinator

Last summer I sent a note to the doc updating him on my blood pressure, and the next thing I heard, he'd electronically sent a prescription change to my nearby Walgreen's, and it was ready to pick up. No need to get a call back from the doctor, etc. And since it's secure email inside their system, it's outside the reach of the Internet snoopers.

But that freedom brings responsibility: if you choose to look into that section, you have to be careful about what you read – just as if you were opening your folder in the doctor's office. I got scared (briefly) about something I read one weekend, left an email for my oncologist, and got it cleared up.

Of course that also requires doctors who are very open – it requires two-way trust and open communication, and doctors who are willing to take what may sometimes be a lot of questions between appointments.

May 22, 2007

I'm going to be quoted in Beth Israel Deaconess's annual report for 2007. It's in a section on Patient Experience, and I'm quoted regarding my love of PatientSite. "Patient Experience" is this hospital's implementation of a business best practice that's vitally important these days but ignored by too many companies, especially those in healthcare.

In general, it's called Customer Experience, and it encompasses every single detail of whether your company is great to deal with or is a royal pain in the patoot. It's been a recognized topic in IT companies for years. Frequently, in IT the issue shows up on the website: is the company's web site great or stinky? (For years some managers resisted upgrading their website, but those managers

> "There's been a paradigm shift: Dr Welby has left the building. What used to be a one-way street is now a two-way street."
>
> — Elizabeth Cohen, Senior Medical Correspondent for CNN (private correspondence)

were tacitly saying they didn't care whether their company was good to deal with.)

I think BID's been pretty fanatical about the total customer (patient) experience for years. For instance, on their appointment reminder letters, the map on the back beats the crap out of the usual. (It's not without faults, but clearly someone sat down and thought about "What can we do to make this a good experience?") The same thinking apparently pervades the design of their new computer systems: "How can we use these systems to make it better to be a BID patient than it has been?" (I haven't been in on those meetings, but the results make it apparent.)

PatientSite is one result. When I log in, I can get results of lab tests, or send a private email to my physician (without using Internet email programs, all of which are vulnerable to snoops and corporate hackers). I can request appointments (and see my doctor's availability calendar), I can request prescriptions. And I can do all of that 24/7, instead of waiting for "Our normal business hours are...." Often, I get a (confidential) reply from my doctor before the next morning. Now, isn't that a better idea ... a better patient experience? (Beth Israel Deaconess isn't the only one who does these things, but they are in a leadership role, and they have technical awards for other behind-the-scenes developments.)

There's one more aspect whose value is hard to give a score to, but it's meant the world to my family recently.

I'm not a medical professional, so there's a limit to how much value I get from an online lab result. Both my wife and my sister in Maryland know much more about such things. So I gave them my PatientSite login, and now either of them can read my lab reports, pathology reports (from a biopsy), scan results, etc., and see if there's anything that catches their eye for further discussion. Imagine trying to do that if the lab report is in a folder in someone's office!

The beauty of all this is that it lets me get more information, even as doctors' time is being squeezed more and more. They do it by just opening the doors so I can see more of my own information.

It takes work for a company (including a hospital) to develop this kind of customer-centered software, but when the rubber hits the road in my real-world case, it makes a real-world difference. That's why when they came looking for testimonials, I raised my hand.

Chapter 6: First Round of Interleukin

April 2 - April 23, 2007

Monday, April 2, 2007 10:58 AM

I gotta say, this place is cool. I'm in the "solarium" (rainy day room) – they have public computers and supposedly they have laptops to take to your room to jack into their DSL connectors. Free DVD/video and CD/tape players in your room, and room service (real cooking, to order, anytime you call down) instead of the usual hospital food.

The people I've met so far are really great – really beyond the norm. Every single one of them has an aura of warmth and welcoming.

Monday, April 2, 2007 12:52 PM

Hi all, well the surgeon is finally here!! We were talking about using "Go Mets" as a slogan. The surgeon suggested we put "Dice the Mets" (for our new pitcher Dice-K). Sounds like a nice t-shirt logo. Only a surgeon could have thought that up! First treatment will be 3pm this pm. All is well so far. Ginny

Monday, April 2, 2007 5:22 PM

I AM ANNOYED!

My last-final-check blood work came back saying that I'm more anemic than I was last week, so before we start the treatment, they're giving me two units of blood. This takes several hours (including everything they have to check) so the treatment's postponed until the morning.

I am (again) tired of finding out one more thing after another to cope with. And, at the same time, while Mr. Annoyance is shouting at the microphone, backstage I'm glad these people know what they're doing and know what to check for, to avoid disasters. And I'm secretly glad I'll be getting a good long night's sleep, which I didn't get last night.

Current plan now is that the treatment will start at 7am.

Thanks to Ginny for insisting that I write this myself, because I didn't want to, because I was being Mister Poopyhead.

Can you tell I'm impatient?

And yes I've been thinking of all of you, as I said I would. Be with me.

Tuesday, April 3, 2007 10:40 AM

Fabulous night of rest, both for me and for Ginny on her cot beside me.

The two units of blood didn't bring the hemoglobin up far enough: needs to be 10, was 8.8, is now 9.8. So they're giving me another unit this morning.

When the docs did their rounds this morning, they said presuming this 3rd unit of blood brings it up above 10, we'll be moving ahead with the whole plan, one day later than scheduled: We'll start at 3pm today and probably go home Monday, not Sunday.

Tuesday, April 3, 2007 6:26 PM

It's official. I am an HDIL-2 user. The battle is joined.

I had my first dose, and my reponse so far is absolutely characteristic.

- felt fine at first

- @90 min I got up to go to the rest room, felt a cool breeze, and got into a good dose of "rigoring" (rye-gor-ing) – shakes for no apparent reason. Treatment is delightful: lie down and be covered with more and more warm blankets. mmmm. But this isn't just any shakes – this was a half hour or more of good solid shaking even when I wasn't cold. Fortunately, not uncomfortable.

- @ 3 hrs, a cough turned into vomiting
- Everything feels just fine now. No big deal, this time!

Wednesday, April 4, 2007 9:53 AM

Well, so far I'm not "beat to hell" by side effects, as I had advertised! I've had some mild effects, but mostly things are mostly okay.

Last night's 11pm dose had no problems – I went right back to sleep.

This morning's 7am dose had no problem, until (an hour later) I started eating my hearty breakfast. That didn't last long, and then it passed and everything's fine.

I do have the first signs of Capillary Leak Syndrome, a common side effect that causes some weight gain and ruddiness in complexion.

So, so far so good on the outside – let's hope the inner game is going as well!

Wednesday, April 4, 2007 4:47 PM

Today's 3pm dose has brought a new (common) side effect: aching joints and bones all over everywhere. Not severe or unbearable yet; staff gave me Oxycodone for it.

No nausea, no chills this afternoon.

Yesterday when I coughed it sometimes caused a "needle going in" response, in the belly, near the incision area. Today it changed to a sense of being cut in that same spot. Dr. Wagner, the surgeon, came in today and said some patients do have that for another week or two. The Oxycodone and Tylenol seem to be managing it, when they don't run out!

So today basically I have symptoms of treatment and no new symptoms of cancer, and that's what we want.

Thursday, April 5, 2007 10:14 AM

Mornin' all! I'm feeling great today. I'm just about ready to join the ranks of those who say the rumors about side effects are overblown, at least for me. I've had no misery at all. Some discomforts, but no misery.

I had another restless night, which is not uncommon for me when I'm alone. (Ginny went home last night to get in a couple of days of work Thur-Fri.) But restlessness is also a potential early warning flag for a neurotoxicity side effect, which can lead to hallucinations and more; so for today's morning dose they're watching me closely. No problems so far.

The common itchiness side effect is building up, slowly, but isn't yet an annoyance. I have plenty of lotions if need be.

I'm in great shape for calls and emails and, on rare occasions, MAYBE a small visit. But those are subject to change.

Thanks for all your support!

Friday, April 6, 2007 9:01 AM

Tired today. All health signs are great, but after the 11pm dose last night I couldn't get to sleep. So I'm going to try to nap as much as possible today.

Last night I didn't have the restlessness of the previous night. Just couldn't get back to sleep.

It's hard to believe but I've completed 9 doses already, and I've got the green light for #10 this afternoon.

I know I've said that the norm for a full set is 12, but it's actually 14. I'm looking good to complete the whole set, 11pm Saturday, then rest Sunday and go home Monday.

Dave

p.s. Thanks for the gift basket from ol' dorm buddy Micky DuPree. It continues to amaze me, how many of you are out there listening!

Saturday, April 7, 2007 10:47 AM

Good Morning friends and family, Ginny here.

It is Saturday morning and our Dave is beat! He finally has had the promised nasty side effects of his treatment. His digestive tract is protesting in its entirety. He said he hadn't eaten in 2 days...water comes up...however, he is the ONLY patient on the floor that completed 12 doses of HDIL-2! The doc gave him a symbolic gold star and decided he had enough for this round...YAH. Now we go on the week of recovery. He will stay in the hospital until Monday a.m...40 hours after the last dose to make sure his heart works OK. No hallucinations, just fatigue and GI symptoms. He has gained some "water weight" but not like I envisioned. His skin is a little itchy, but no "snowstorms" yet. One of the promised side effects is lots and lots of flaky skin.

I'll be checking in with you for the next few days while Dave catches up on sleep and energy.

I guess that is all for now. Thank you again for all the well wishes and love you have sent. Happy Easter everyone. Ginny (and Dave)

Saturday, April 7, 2007 11:34 AM

Hi, I just had another thought about how some of you might be able to help. Our house in Minnesota is still unsold. We just listed it again after renting it all winter. If anybody knows anyone that would like to buy a really nice house, let us know. It would take a BIG burden off us if could be sold.

Thanks, Ginny

Sunday, April 8, 2007 11:28 AM

Hi deB fans, it is Ginny signing in again. Dave had a great night's sleep with the help of Benadryl for his increasingly itchy skin. He has a dry cottony mouth while his mouth skin sloughs and there is increasing evidence of the predicted "snow storm" on his outer skin layer. The Doc stopped in and said the first 24 hours after

IL-2 stops is the worst. He will probably spend Easter Sunday sleeping. He is groggy and he can't speak well because of the condition of his mouth. This uncomfortable period should end in the next few days....then we can do it all over again! Hopefully next time there won't be so many infusions. The nurse said the goal is 18-24. Time will tell.

I hope all of you are enjoying the renewal that spring brings. The good thing about spring snow storms is they don't stay with us very long.

We will think about that summer time CaringBridge reunion. It would be great to meet all of you!

If any of you nearby friends would like to stay with Dave next Friday while I go to work it would be great.

Again thanks for all your support, Ginny

Sunday, April 8, 2007 1:16 PM

A quick note from me myself this time – yes, I'm all beat up, tired as can be, into the dry-everything phase. Very glad to be (apparently) out of the total digestive shutdown phase, and VERY eager to get out of the very dry mouth phase.

That's all for now. I continue to be uplifted and so heartened by all your support.

Love,

Dave

Monday, April 9, 2007 8:05 PM

Hi everyone, Dave and I made it home from the hospital today. A busy time getting all his meds organized (8, I think) when to give them etc., getting unpacked and taking a shower after 3 days in the hospital, getting clothes washed etc. My wonderful children came over and cleaned house for us while we were gone. Dave is still working on keeping water and jello down. Coughing is still an issue. Itchy skin has subsided. He really looks forward to the simple experience of a spoonful of jello or a sip of water without coughing.

Thank you for the incredible stream of wonderful cards and letters that keep coming. Keep praying and hoping it "ain't over yet" (deB).

Thanks to Sandy for her incredibly generous offer to take care of Dave this week while I am at work.

Ginny

Monday, April 9, 2007 9:55 PM

Dave here – some quick points – it's great to be back home and so great to no longer have bags of immunochemicals infused in me at 3pm, 11pm, and 7am, and blood samples taken from me every few hours. It's so great that when I go to the john I no longer have to tote my IV pole with me. etc. What a relief! At the same time I'm acutely aware that this isn't even half over yet: Tuesday we go back in for another week, and then a week later there's the big scan, and a week after THAT the docs say whether we got any results. So we must keep on, and we ask you to keep sending all your thoughts and prayers and intentions. We intend to keep creating insanely unreasonable results with all of your support. Find the best possible care, learn as much as we can, and above all, keep a clear mind and a strong mental attitude. You continue to support us in too many ways to count. Bless you!

Tuesday, April 10, 2007 9:10 PM

Hi all, Dave is lacking energy today. Today is his first day of complete rest in weeks. He enjoyed sitting in our new reclining chair. It was MUCH more comfortable than trying to sit up in bed. He watched the Red Sox wallop Seattle...yeah! He actually ate some solid food today and kept it down. Not much, mind you...a little at a time. He insists that I include this:

> "Words can't begin to describe how much a caregiver
> provides in a situation like this. I can't fathom where

someone like me would be without someone like Ginny. Thanks so much to each of you who has given care in a similar situation. Without you we would be desperate."

I actually woke up and found he had made his way to the living room by himself so I could sleep. His way of taking care of me.

Ginny

Wednesday, April 11, 2007 10:37 PM

As planned, today was a day of rest – for me, anyway. Ginny continues being a fountain of generosity and hard work, and tomorrow Sandy takes over, while Ginny goes to work.

For those of you who don't know, Sandy is my first wife, a wonderful person, former clinical intensive care nurse at Mass General, and now involved in cardiac research there.

As you might imagine, my gratitude for her assistance and generosity in this is beyond words. I'm blessed to have people like this supporting me. (To make a long story short, caring for me at this moment is not just a matter of making a sandwich now and then.)

Finally, today I got another 6 cards in the mail from you. You continue to amaze me, and the thoughts you send my way truly give me strength to be with this situation and be fully effective, whatever form that takes.

Love,

Dave

Friday, April 13, 2007 5:13 PM

For the past two days I've been cared for superbly by Sandy, my first wife. She used flex time from work to come stay overnight and be a terrific caregiver for two full days. In addition to all the "doing" she did for me (tending to all kinds of things), her perceptiveness had her notice when I was getting anxious about things, before I even realized it, so we could intervene appropriately.

I'm so blessed. And I mean, truly, no matter what your point of view regarding religion, no matter what the word means to you, I am blessed.

We called the hospital a couple of times to check on specific items yesterday and today, spoke with Spectacular Nurse Megan, and learned that it sounds like everything's going according to plan. Similarly when Kendra the research coordinator called to confirm next week's schedule I said the past couple of days had been yucky and she said "Yup – I don't even TRY to call before Thursday."

It's amazing to me that it's possible to take a complex system like the human body, give it a whacking stiff treatment like this high-dosage Interleukin, and be able to predict with such regularity what's going to happen when.

Beyond the technical skill aspect of it, there's the people aspect: it means SO much to me that I can reach the specific people who've been caring for me and get their reading. I have the experience of still being in their care.

Sunday, April 15, 2007 11:44 PM

PROGRESS

Ginny observes that I spent a lot of energy Saturday. Did some non-trivial business at the bank, got a pesky slow leak fixed at Sullivan Tire, made my own dinner (just freezer stuff, but it's more than I've been doing). And today we played cards for the first time in weeks.

AS TIME GOES BY (and appetite returns)

One's sense of time is a funny thing. I came home from Week 1 last Monday. In these 6 days I went through phases of violent indigestion, patchy sleep, total lack of energy, restoration, and finally this weekend the return of a voracious appetite, eating full servings of chicken piccata, ice cream, ravioli, puddings, nachos, cheesecake... all today.

It's unfathomable to me that all these phases happened in just 6 days. Seems like weeks.

NEXT STEPS

- Tuesday 4/17 thru Monday 4/23: in hospital for week 2 of HDIL-2

- Monday 4/23: Appt with orthopedic surgeon to re-assess left femur. Can I walk again without a walker??

- Monday 4/23 – Sunday 4/30: repeat this past week's recuperation

- Monday 5/14: CAT scans to see how the mets have responded to HDIL-2

- Thursday 5/18: Hospital's tumor board reviews my case

- Monday 5/21: Meet with oncologists to get results of scan and next steps

Tuesday, April 17, 2007 11:27 PM

We're underway for week 2.

I've just had my second dose. The first was the same as 2 weeks ago: no noticeable effects except chills, which responded well to warm blankets and never came back. Had a great dinner, watched the Sox game, ready for bed.

Good to hear from you, Kate. You mention "MS is getting boring." Cool! A couple of months ago I posted that there's increasing news of kidney cancer treatments that stop the disease from progressing, so it becomes a chronic condition to manage, not a death threat. I'm wide open to the idea of this kidney cancer becoming "boring" like your MS!

p.s. Hot news: Monique Doyle Spencer, author of *The Courage Muscle* (below), plans to drop by and meet me! What fun WE can have!

Laugh, Sing, and Eat Like a Pig

Thursday, April 19, 2007 8:51 PM

Hiatus! After 3 doses (ending Wednesday morning), I had one of the most common Interleukin side effects: my blood pressure plummeted (at one point down to 69/39). This is one of the biggie side effects that they watch for, and when it happens, they jump in and intervene big-time.

The ability to handle this effectively, outside an ICU, is apparently one of the big advances in recent years. Needless to say, I'm grateful.

The intervention is that I got hooked up to a snazzy new machine that automatically checks BP every 15 minutes and buzzes the station if it's below target; and I got an additional med, which got changed to something stronger, then changed back.

We skipped three doses of Interleukin so far (a full day), waiting for the BP to settle down. Right now it looks like tonight's 11pm dose has a good chance – but, safety first.

Monique (see below) visited me today! We hit it off instantly. (She brought me a sheet of temporary Red Sox tattoos, and we had a good time dreaming up mischievous places they could be placed, inside a pajama top, to raise eyebrows.)

I have a feeling we're going to have a lot of fun as time goes by.

♦　　♦　　♦

Finally, I had an unexpected visitor. Around suppertime, dressed in apron and hair net, in walked Paul Levy, CEO of the place. It turns out he's job-shadowing Food Service tonight, and was out delivering meals. From the grin on his face, he was lovin' it.

Here's hopin' my BP cooperates and I get my 11pm dose and we go back on the full protocol!

Friday, April 20, 2007 4:11 AM

A DOSE IN THE WEE HOURS

1. The BP still misbehaved, but slowly got to where it belongs. So

I got my next dose at 3:30 a.m. E.T. So I'll be off-schedule for the rest of the stay (unless we skip another dose and sync up again).

So I've now had 16 doses total, which is great.

2. Tonight, having no interest in sleep, I've been reading Monique's "The Courage Muscle," and it's a much better book than I'd even expected. In addition to its funny often-bratty humor, it has a lot of real-world practical advice. I recommend, nay urge, that everyone facing cancer take a look at this book. It's a quick easy read, too.

—Well, supernurse Megan finally coaxed me in the direction of taking something to sleep, and I agreed. Bye for now.

Saturday, April 21, 2007 9:23 AM

DOSE 17, AT LAST!

After my previous entry, my BP just would not cooperate (and the medics here insisted on being safe), so dose 17 of Interleukin-2 has just started, some 29 hours after dose 16.

I must say that it was wonderful to spend an entire day with no digestive symptoms at all! And I got a complete night of solid sleep. What a GREAT idea!

◆　　◆　　◆

Hey, wanna know how crazy my sister Suede is? Yesterday afternoon she phoned from Logan airport in Boston, en route to her next gig, and said, "Hey, I got to the airport way early – do you have time for me to cab to your hospital for a half hour visit?" And she did.

WAITING FOR NEWS: Patience required

On Friday I got an answer to a question that's been bugging me: is there a connection between my final outcome and my apparent symptoms after Week 1 of treatment?

I asked because the lump on my arm was bigger at the start of week 2, which left me wondering "Is this stuff not working???"

The answer is that there's no connection. Kidney cancer is an immune system disease with immune system treatment, and that's very different from most other treatments. You don't necessarily see the results until well after the treatment's been delivered.

So, as much as I like to watch data and get updates in real time, I'm outa luck on this score: I just gotta be a patient patient!

Sunday, April 22, 2007 9:27 AM

And a fine top o' the morrrnin' to ye!

It looks like the treatments are finished for this go-round. My BP continued to misbehave so I didn't get a sixth dose of IL-2 this time, so the total is 5 doses this week, 17 for the 2 weeks.

I expressed disappointment to excellent nurse Gretchen and she said not to worry, she's seen patients get only 6/week and still have a good response.

And, the GREAT news (I realized) is that with the much smaller dose, I'm probably going to have a much easier recovery. My digestive symptoms seem to have already cleared (hooRAY, and Ginny agrees) and I've gained half as much water weight and I have no "water balloon ankles."

♦   ♦   ♦

A note about the value of your support: The BP machine automatically takes a reading every 15 minutes, round the clock. This sometimes wakes me up. One more time I want to repeat that when I'm lying in the hospital bed in the wee hours, I do think of your support, and it makes a difference.

Monday, April 23, 2007 3:24 PM

We're home. I woke up at 4am for the daily lab samples, and for some reason I was awake for good. Once again, today I do NOT feel like I have cancer. Given all the inconsistencies one could have in life, this is one that I endorse. :-)

Got discharged from the IL-2 unit early. Ginny once again deserves an enormous amount of acknowledgement for all the work she did gathering and packing all our belongings and toting them to the car.

We visited the orthopod (bone doc) and got new x-rays and a brief meeting. The femur looks cautiously optimistic. Bottom line, it'll be several months before I might be able to walk unassisted again, maybe longer. But there's a good chance the leg will heal itself without surgery.

The left forearm (a much less important item) is worse but not a huge problem, nor a priority in the treatment plan (it's painless).

Driving home today, I got one of those nutso ideas in my head and called the office and we ended up meeting Ed & Marc for lunch. I might have acted a bit manic at times (who, ME?), but it was great to see them and talk about everything that's been going on in my life and at the office.

And if any of you say "Why are you even THINKING about work??", I say "Find work you love."

And now Ginny and I are off to a great big long-lasting NAP!

Chapter 7: The Web is Changing Healthcare

> We modestly suggest that the tentative conclusions
> below are no more 'anti-doctor' or 'anti-medicine' than
> the conclusions of Copernicus and Galileo were anti-
> astronomer.
>
> – e-Patients White Paper, "Seven Preliminary
> Conclusions," Chapter 2 (*see Appendix*)

Many people, clinicians and lay alike, worry about the trust-worthiness of information on the web. My own experience tells me that online patient communities can provide information that is critical for your health and that is available nowhere else. But as everyone knows, there's also a lot of crap out there. The question is, how do we learn the difference?

Dr. Sands talks about getting used to the idea of "knowledge symmetry" – the new reality that patients can bring legitimate information to the table that the physician might not have seen. And he counsels his colleagues to coach patients: suggest good websites, teach them how to tell good from bad, etc.

I look at it this way: The Pew Internet and American Life Project reported in June 2009 that 61% of adults seek health information online. Are we going to tell them not to (that's absurd), or will we empower, educate, and enable them?

Here are some post-cancer blog posts from my personal pathway as I got to know this issue.

Thursday, February 7, 2008

Web 2.0 means "we get to say."

My previous post mentions "2.0" stuff. I've been dealing with this subject at work for the past year, but I know a lot of you have only recently heard this "buzzword" buzzing around like an annoying gnat that keeps getting in your ear, making it hard to think.

Some of the key aspects of Web 2.0 for the engaged patient are:

- blogs
- wikis (Wikipedia is just one example)
- social networks
- social bookmarks.

The big deal about all this is "user generated content" (UGC). See, in the early days of the web (now known as Web 1.0), the web was read-only: all web "content" (the stuff you read or view) was created by people who had access to a web server and knew all the geeky stuff you needed for hand coding a web page.

In contrast to that, today we can create content: Look, I'm sitting here right now, blogging about whatever I want – just as if I could conceive and write a book and get it printed and have it appear in every library in the world, instantly. (Because it IS, right now, available on every computer in the world that has an Internet connection, including my iPod Touch.)

This that you're reading, right here, is user-generated content.

And the big thing about THAT is that it's enabled us to spout our opinions, for instance rating books on Amazon or even posting our own book reviews, as short or as long as we want.

What this means in the world of e-patients is that we ourselves get to talk about anything we want; instead of reading only what a magazine editor thinks we want (or need to know), we ourselves get to start any discussion we want and take it anywhere we want.

You could put it this way: Web 2.0 means we get to say. We get to say whatever we want, and we even get to say what gets talked about.

This is a core principle cited in the e-patients white paper, which you really should read.

Laugh, Sing, and Eat Like a Pig

Sunday, February 10, 2008

An e-patient writes in Newsweek.com

Newsweek.com has published "A Healing Blog," a well-written article by the amazing Amy Tenderich, author of DiabetesMine (www.diabetesmine.com) , a prize-winning diabetes blog. Here's a perfect e-patient snip from her article:

> I'm just astounded to think that one sick mom in California can reach out to so many fellow patients, create a community, and actually turn the whole thing into a business.

Amy's story illustrates a major aspect of the e-patient movement: that if patients (the consumers of healthcare) get to start conversations and other patients get to take those conversations wherever they want, the most useful conversations will thrive, and all of us – consumers and providers alike – will benefit.

Chapter 2 of the e-patients White Paper (see Appendix) lists seven principles of patient-driven healthcare. Amy's article illustrates three of the seven:

#1. E-patients have become valuable healthcare resources and providers should recognize them as such.

#3. We have underestimated patients' ability to provide useful online resources.

#7. The most effective way to improve healthcare is to make it more collaborative.

Plus, it quietly suggests support for a fourth:

#4. We have overestimated the hazards of imperfect online health information.

#4 doesn't say there are no hazards – you and I need to be smart consumers, same as if we're buying a car or a camera. It says that those risks are manageable: all of us (patients and providers alike) can publicly holler "BS!" when we see it. In the process, we learn to find trusted resources – like Amy's blog.

Welcome, Amy! Keep spreading the word, and keep in touch.

Wednesday, March 5, 2008

"Succeeding in online health" lunch meeting

The Mass. Technology Leadership Council is (as I type this) having a "lunch and learn" session titled "Patient, Heal Thyself: How to Succeed with Online Consumer Health Sites." When I first read the title, I heard "How to make a great online consumer health site," but hey, it's a high-tech business lunch, so in fact it's about how to make a buck at it.

That's fine with me – the "helping people save their butts" community can use some infusions of cash, as investors take advantage of the reality that billions of people are entering the phase of life where they get serious illness and want to have their butts saved. Build great, useful online health resources, and the world will improve.

Here's a clue, investors: to build success, don't sit in a conference room figuring out what someone would want, and do NOT emulate the many web sites that say "Here is what we believe you should want to know." Just ask patients what they want to talk about.

I'm not being anti-establishment here, I'm being businesslike. Peer-reviewed medical journals may be full of reproducible experimental results, but (a) they may not answer what people want to ask, and (b) as happened in my cancer, the best current peer-reviewed journal articles may not be useful anymore. Ironically, people whose butts are on the line may find (as I did) that those are not always reliable resources! They are necessary, to be sure, but their content may be obsolete, and they may not even answer the questions people want to ask.

Tom Ferguson MD, founder of the e-Patient Scholars Working Group , felt strongly that we often have it upside down, when we have doctors decide what people need to hear. And as we move into e-health, I think he's right: failure to ask patients "what do you want to hear about?" will be as deadly (business-wise) in online health as it was in any other industry that went through its "railroad" phase. (Can you say "marketing myopia"?)

It's a simple business principle – ordinary consumer market research. *Do not* start by asking the providers what they think we consumers should hear. Use them as a highly valued resource, but don't start by asking them.

A huge part of the discussion (today and elsewhere) concerns "safety" of the information people acquire by researching online. I put "safety" in quotes because it's a big mistake to think that well-vetted certified MD-approved info is the best path to safety: every bit of misleading or useless info I got last year came from well-vetted web sites. The only indication of quality that I found was whether other "consumers" of the information (patients and their families) said the info was reliable.

As I mentioned, I'm writing while attending a meeting on online health services. At one point in the meeting, I stood up and remarked that we all use car ratings guides when we buy a car, and that the same will surely happen with online consumer health info.

John Lester of SecondLife addressed the safety question in a characteristically fun/ny way: "If fire were invented today, there's no way it would get on the market. You'd have to say 'okay, we won't make it too hot, and we'll add warning labels...' If you'd told someone 200 years ago that we'd be roaming around in these things called 'cars' that have hundreds of little controlled explosions of fire every minute, they'd think you're crazy." Amen, bro. Things that seem insanely impractical today may only seem that way because we're two generations too young!

I've always wondered what real use can be made of SecondLife – the classic "is it just a toy?" question. Well, it's so richly experiential that someone has used it to show others what a psychotic hallucination is like. Others are using it for "first response" training. Autistics are using it to develop their social skills.

Kids are using virtual gaming to attack cancer cells – an online manifestation of the well-known practice of visualizations as a way of fighting cancer. (One kid I read about visualized little sharks going through his veins eating cancer cells. Now, I suppose, he could create that happening "in-world," as the SecondLifers say.)

Last weekend at the e-Patient Scholars Working Group retreat, I had the profound privilege of being with Kevin Kelly, co-founding Executive Editor of *Wired* and author of *New Rules of the New Economy*. He blew our minds by pointing out that in 2007 the web became just 5,000 days old.

The first 5,000 days brought web sites, Google, Travelocity, blogs, webcams, Napster, Facebook, SecondLife, and a lot more. Imagine: what will the next 5,000 days bring?

Chapter 8: Returning to Work – Mastering Mobility

April 25 - May 10, 2007

Wednesday, April 25, 2007 6:16 PM

I'm returning to work Tuesday!

Week 2 of HDIL-2 therapy is supposed to have a 2-3 week recovery period. But I'm having no symptoms at all. Maybe that's because I only got 5 doses this time – I dunno. Or, maybe it has something to do with the enormous amounts of support you-all are giving me, or how I'm being about the whole thing, or all of the above.

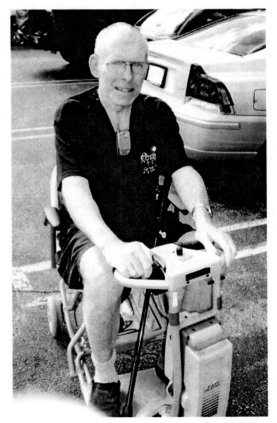

My snazzy Tzora scooter. (These photos were taken in August, as I returned it to the rental place. The short hair is due to a haircut – more on this later.)

But in any case my energy level is great – not even any mid-day naps – and I have no digestive or other symptoms.

It's ironic: we were working on the paperwork to get me approved for short-term disability coverage when I realized "Wait a minute, how exactly am I disabled??" There are 2 answers: I can't walk (millions of people deal with that) and I get winded easily when I have to travel any distance with my uuuugly "platform walker."

"Hm," thinks me; "It's gadget time. Both of those problems would be solved by one o' them snazzy Mobility Scooters that I've seen people use." (The model I had is the Easy Travel Elite from Tzora. Google for "travel scooters" to look for other disassemblable scooters.) To make a long story short, I found a model that one person can disassemble and put in the trunk of a car, and we picked one up on rental. And MAN AM I MOBILE NOW! (I zoom and swivel with grace and aplomb.)

This thing is WELL DESIGNED, unlike most of the "mobility" products I've seen. It was designed & built on a kibbutz in Israel, and has a completely different and efficient design compared to competitors.

It has a super-tight turning radius, maneuvers well in tight hallways, can go up to 4.5mph (faster than most people walk), can go 10.5 miles on a single charge, and has enough power to push open a difficult restroom door ... no small issue, as any wheelchair user will attest.

Re returning to work, my managers are glad to hear it but they're

Folded, the scooter was compact enough to fit in the Prius's trunk.

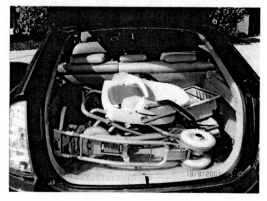

concerned that I not take foolish risks – they say my health & safety are most important. (Ain't that a nice attitude?? And I know they mean it.) First step was to get the oncologist's okay; he said "Sounds reasonable to me – save the disability coverage for later."

Next was that they don't want me making myself work when I'm really not well; we agreed on that. (In a conference call today, Ginny pointed out that she and I were on the go all day today, and I'm going to chorus tonight, and my energy level is still good. And, she said (to my surprise & pleasure), "I haven't seen him this alive in a LONG time.")

Nice. So it's a go.

THRUSH?! ME??

Last week I was tormented for several days with some sort of mouth problem. At first I thought it was just a ton of cracked-lip things, related to dry mouth, a common symptom from the IL-2 and other meds they use. But this was all over my tongue and the inside of my mouth, and eventually it got to the point where it felt like 100 razor cuts in my mouth. (I'm not kidding.)

When I finally told the doctor during rounds one morning, he looked and said "I think you've got thrush!" (A yeast infection, often occurring as a result of being on antibiotics ... normal mouth bacteria ordinarily keep the yeast at bay, and antibiotics can sometimes upset that balance.)

I gather this is more often seen in newborns, but that's what he said. I said, "How do we confirm the diagnosis?" He said "We don't, we just treat it." And indeed, after a couple of doses of some foamy rinse concoction, the "razor cuts" went away. (I'm finishing all of the concoction, as directed, to keep it away.)

DRY SKIN AND PEELING

One last thing...it's normal with HDIL-2 to have all your skin peel off, twice (once per week). After the first week I had some fascinating "snowstorms" – take off your shirt and have a snowstorm of skin flakes (like dandruff) fill the air. Eeuuuw? That's up to you. I was mildly amused.

But this week, again perhaps because of only 5 doses, I'm not having snowstorms – I'm having my skin dry up into flakes while still on my body, and stay there, looking scruffy. This is gross.

It tends to happen all at once in a region, and it can be quite surprising. Like, Monday on the way to lunch with Marc & Ed, I looked in the mirror and discovered that my FACE was suddenly coated with skin flakes. I looked like a ghoul. Fortunately a few minutes of hard work in the men's room resolved (most of) it.

Adventures in cancer therapy. Who knew?

◆　　◆　　◆

It's not in the CaringBridge journal, but once I found that scooter, things moved rapidly. The problem was that it didn't fit easily into the trunk of my Camry Hybrid. So, through a series of marvelous events I traded it in for a shiny new Prius, with its big hatchback.

Monday, April 30, 2007 6:02 PM

Sorry for the five-day gap since my last post – I didn't mean to alarm anyone. Didn't realize it'd been that long!

Caveat: there is no cancer news to report. Everything is just "how life is going." (That's the main reason it's been so long.)

MY BUTT HURTS

Those of you who've spent time in a wheelchair will know what I mean by this. We get TIRED of sitting!

There's an often-used wisecrack (it's on a coffee cup in Mom's kitchen window) that's something like "We're not getting lazy. We're developing powerful muscles that allow us to sit for a very long time without getting tired." I now know this isn't just a joke: My physical therapist gave me a butt-clenching exercise.

My ultimate recourse is where I am right now: The Comfy Chair – the rocker-recliner that takes the load off those muscles and supports me uniformly from head to heel.

NEXT TREATMENT EVENTS

Monday 5/14 – CT scan to see how the HDIL affected the mets

Monday 5/21 – Meet with the treatment team to see what's next.

Monday June 11 & 18 – Another scan and team meeting

If I'm to get another 2-week batch of HDIL, it'll be late summer.

THE RETURN TO NORMALCY CONTINUES

Preparing for the return to work tomorrow, this weekend we collected all of my unopened mail, some dating back to late December (just before this adventure started) and I plowed through almost all of it. Tonight I'll complete the current round of bill payments, and that'll be done for now.

We want to ditch the house in Minnesota, at almost any price. We dropped the price again and had an open house yesterday; we're dropping it again this week. Now that the tenants have moved out, I'll do just about anything to stop the $3000/month carrying costs! (Mortgages, utilities, property tax, mowing.....)

I say it's a good thing when my top concerns are plain old bills and a sore butt.

Tuesday, May 1, 2007 6:46 PM

The first day back at work was great. There was a colorful "Welcome Back Dave" poster at the front door, balloons and garlands in my cubicle, along with a poster signed by many people, and a big *delicious* Welcome Back Dave cake at lunch.

Everyone was terrific.

Driving into the parking lot was as if I'd never left. (Well, it WAS only 8 weeks ago.)

Friend Bill Roberts sent a note today saying "Methinks this is a majorly good ting." I agree.

Oh, btw, my scooter skills need more honing – I did a bit more wall-banging than desired in the cubicle farm. ;->

◆   ◆   ◆

Folks, re the recent 5-day gap between messages: that may happen again - don't worry. If anything drastic befell me, Ginny would be here telling you. If there's no news here, it's because life is being blissfully unexciting. :)

Tuesday, May 1, 2007 7:46 PM

This is my second post tonight.

Although my spirit, mind, and body are feeling terrific at the moment, I am aware (and I'd like you to be aware) that it ain't over, and I invite you to join me in focusing on what comes next.

First, I presume that there is more curing to be done on the mets throughout my body. They may not be acting up or producing symptoms at the moment but the HDIL team basically said nobody becomes "NED" (No Evidence of Disease) clean on one round of HDIL. So there's more work to do.

The other thing has more immediate impact: two bone mets continue to give challenges. The femur seems stable but it has a long way to go until it's healed, and until then I'm hobbled in my mobility and at risk of fracture.

I have a bigger annoyance and risk with my left forearm. The x-ray a week ago showed that it's worse, and I said it's not painful; but now it is becoming mildly painful, a trend that I want to clear up. And what the x-ray showed is that there's been significant erosion of that bone. I can't put much load on it now (pulling or pushing) and if it erodes more it'll eventually break.

The doc says the bone can fully repair itself, but that will not start until that tumor (that bone met) is completely dead. And that's not happening – if anything that met is growing. You can feel it from the outside – like an egg or a golf ball buried in the arm.

So for those of you who focus curative energy on things, my primary request tonight is that we visualize and create a healthy, intact, pure, clean, fully natural left forearm.

Tumors can die rapidly. And remember, kidney cancer and melanoma are the cancers with the highest rate of spontaneous remission, aka self-cure.

I am fully in the game of creating this outcome, and I invite you to join me.

Thursday, May 3, 2007 6:54 PM

Well, three days into it, work is going great.

It's so funny – the people at work are intrigued and amused by my scooter, and I'm sure not gonna stop 'em! And they're so great, 15-20 of them signed up for the list to come down and help me get the scooter out of the car in the morning. Great bunch of people.

It's SO good to have something on the calendar besides hospital visits for scans and treatments!

Mind you, I do get tired working, even tho all I do is desk-sit. I imagine it'll improve – I'm VERY out of practice at responding to an alarm clock!

But it's a good tired, not "lord am I beat" or exhausted or dead to the world. To the contrary, I realized that the yawns I have now are *delicious*: I told Ginny it feels like the kind of g.r.e.a.t ... b.i.g ... y.a.w.n that little babies do. Wonderful.

And some days, like yesterday, I come home and fall into The Comfy Chair and just watch a whole Red Sox game, snoozing when I snooze.

◆　◆　◆

Yesterday was the first time since March 2 that Ginny's had a day at home, alone, without me. Yay for her!

DEPT OF TRANSPORTATION

The Prius reports that for its first 436 miles, it's averaging 51.8 mpg. This too is good. The scooter cubicle-banging is improving, and I can now zip into the elevator in reverse, making it much easier to exit in a crowd. Ah, gadgets.

At the other end of the scale, a college friend is riding his bicycle (right now) from home in Berkeley to Boston for our 35th reunion a month from now. His blog has some breathtaking writing and photos. Biking 100+ miles a day, for a month? Hard work. He said he might post something about me tonight (overnight) and similarities in our journeys.

ENTERTAINMENT

Sister Suede has booked herself into a great venue near here for the night of Saturday July 28. Seriously, if you're near Boston or NH, please plan to attend – it is sure to be a highly spiritual and rollicking evening. Tupelo Music Hall, Londonderry, NH. She says after this group (us here) has bought tickets, her peeps from around New England and the US will fill whatever seats remain. (Yes, she has people who fly across the country to see her.) So let's get in while we can. I would *so* love to see every one of you.

Sunday, May 6, 2007 10:53 PM

A busy weekend, busy with ordinary things: shopping, cleaning and such.

We continue to be moved by the support people give us. Today Ginny's cousin Bob (a builder/remodeler) and wife Louise came over and seriously upgraded our garage landing (adding a ramp) to make it easier for me to get in and out of the house. They put in hours of skilled work.

One more thing – I think I haven't said enough here to acknowledge how fortunate I've been to have access to such excellent medical care. Thanks to everyone who was ever involved in developing these treatments!

And thanks to all of you for your support of the mental and spiritual aspect.

Tuesday, May 8, 2007 8:32 PM

Work continues to go well. Today I took an hour nap, and stayed an hour late to make up for it. I've been put in charge of the relationship with our newly hired PR firm, which is a bunch of very good, stimulating people. Really looking forward to producing results with them!

Today I phoned "my" unit in the hospital and left them a bulletin board message about how well things are going. Funny, it seems like ages ago that I was in the hospital, but it was only two weeks ago.

Next Monday I go back for the CAT scans that will show the remaining size of all the mets. On the kidney cancer mailing list, people talk about something called "scanxiety" as they approach these scans. I can understand that. I don't feel overtly anxious, but I must say, I sure hope the scans show that my inner body is doing as well as I feel on the outside! And I won't know the outcome of the scans until our team meeting a week later ... so all there is to do is relax, chill, meditate, visualize.

♦   ♦   ♦

The Prius continues to please me: today the dashboard says the current tank is running at 53.4 mpg.

♦   ♦   ♦

And finally, in the category of Make Dave Laugh, in recent days I've been getting GREAT results from my Calvin & Hobbes books, and from watching "Whose Line Is It Anyway." The creator of that cartoon strip, and the people on that show, are all MANIACS. It's clearly not possible to do what they do.

And that too is a good state of mind: to be in the presence of things that clearly aren't possible but are happening nonetheless. It stretches one's concept of what's possible for a human being.

Tuesday, May 8, 2007 9:27 PM

p.s. to tonight's posting:

I keep forgetting to mention that this experience seems to have given me two good physical effects that are persisting:

1. For the first time in 10 years, my blood pressure is fine without medication. (It dropped 30 points when the bad kidney was removed.)

2. Compared to the last 20 years, my weight is down 30 pounds (healthily). I'm within 11 pounds of my ideal weight, and my body mass index is 25.9, vs. a desired range of 18-25.

Mind you, I wouldn't recommend cancer as a way to ACHIEVE these results. :-) But what's so is so, and I like it!

Thursday, May 10, 2007 10:01 PM

I left work early today, making good on my promise not to push myself unwisely: I felt run-down, so I left, and had a relaxing afternoon at home.

LONG NOTE OF TECHNICAL NEWS

I learned some new info today about developments in predicting who'll have a good response to IL-2 (the treatment I'm getting). Caveat: if you're not interested in nuts & bolts details, the rest of this post will bore you.

As I've said before, only about 20% of people who receive IL-2 have any response. The treatment is risky and expensive, so doctors would much rather only give it to people it will help. The problem is that they don't yet know how to predict that. So there's a lot of work going on, to try to uncover what factors predict success.

Today I learned about three factors that were new to me. (Only one is well established and accepted yet, but it's all fascinating to me.) Ginny found an article on Medscape about Interleukin-2, with links to other articles, covering two factors I hadn't heard about. One is a "transmembrane protein that may be associated with progression [of the disease] and survival." It's called carbonic anhydrase IX (CAIX), and if it responds strongly to a certain stain, it seems to predict success with IL-2. (I say "seems" because it's not been studied enough to be accepted.)

Of course :-), I wrote to my oncology team asking where I sit on the CAIX staining scale. The score to beat is 85%. For the chemically oriented, there's a brief article about the family of carbonic anhydrase enzymes in Wikipedia. CAIX is #9, hence the IX.

The other factor is "pathology and morphology": certain factors in cell type and structure of the tumor. If your cell type is clear cell RCC (mine is), and the tumor cells have a strongly alveolar structure (a nice neat cluster), you're in a good risk group regarding IL-2. If the structure is 2 other types, you're in an intermediate risk group. And if it's something else, you're in the high risk group.

Here's the big thing: Of the 27 people who responded to IL-2, *26* were in the good risk group, or they were in the intermediate risk group and had a favorable CAIX score (>85%). Hear that?? 26 out of 27 responders were in those groups! So guess where I want to be. And so of course when I wrote to my team, I also asked them about my morphology.

Finally, another assessment scale ("SANI") has been developed to assess risk and recommend treatment, for people (like me) who have a nephrectomy followed by Interleukin. On that scale, I'm in the intermediate risk group, with above-average survival and chance of response. That's a big step up from the view I had 4 months ago, in which I was in the group with the worst outlook!

Of course, all of this is just a mind game: what's so is so, whether or not I know it, and reality doesn't change when new information comes to my attention. But I'm happy to look for any evidence that reinforces my experience that I'm healing!

Chapter 9: Whose Cancer Is It, Anyway?

The power of how we choose to view life

Throughout this story a recurring theme is the power of the mind: a strong mental attitude and maintaining clear consciousness, so that our human mental concerns don't make things worse than they are. I'd like to take a break from the storyline to present a number of posts, from CaringBridge and afterward, that express this.

There's no way to know with certainty how strong a role attitude played in my outcome, but I can say with certainty that my experience of the illness was optimized by my choice not to get wrapped up in imaginary, negative thoughts.

I think this is important for cancer patients to realize. The truth is that even if the odds are bad, you have no way of knowing with certainty what your outcome will be, so don't make it worse than it is. And as I said in the Hope chapter, this was driven home when my oncologist, no New Age hippie, said, "You have an incredible life force."

I can't guarantee you a thing, but speaking as one patient who made the journey, I recommend having as clear a mind and as strong an attitude as you want. I'm personally confident about one thing: if you delude yourself about reality, or if you make up misery that's perhaps imaginary, you will dilute your ability to deal with reality. And that will squander whatever life force you have.

Here are a series of posts from CaringBridge, and later blog posts, reflecting on all this. One of the earliest thoughts was the profound question, "Whose cancer is it, anyway? Who grew this thing?"

Laugh, Sing, and Eat Like a Pig

Saturday, February 10, 2007 [6 weeks after the x-ray]

What do we name the tumor?

Okay, you know me: I'm a brat about just about everything. I heard that some people name their cancer and talk to it. So I've been (idly) wondering what to name this thing. Nothing normal, that's for sure – nothing like "Frank." I want it to be something really disrespectful, something that would make it curl up in shame and just get out of town. What to call it... it's a kidney cancer; call it "Kid Can"? Naaah. "KC"? Bleah.

Thursday I had dinner with daughter Lindsey and she got That Look in her eye. She looked off to the side and came back with "How about Reeni? For renal cell carcinoma?" I kinda like it – it suggests a sneering "Neener neener neener, Reeni is a wiener."

Monday, February 19, 2007 10:30 PM

I'm going to stick my neck out here about how to relate to the cancer inside me.

About ten days ago I posted about coming up with an insulting name for the cancer, something to make it shrivel up and get out of town.

A few days later, Sister Suede raised a thought I've heard (rarely) from others, that there might be another way to look at it: that the cancer is actually part of me (which it is – homegrown by Yours Truly), and it's something to have a different sort of relationship with.

I've thought about it since then, and I want to explore this. Please play along for a minute.

♦   ♦   ♦

All these tumor cells are actually part of me, from me, created by my body.

My rewording of Suede's observation is that there's no integrity in viewing it as something foreign. It's a mistake, and will surely leave me with no power to be effective in relating to it.

So I'm looking for a way to acknowledge that this is actually part of me. It's a part that may be working against me, and a part of me that I may not like; but if I don't grant what's so, or if I make it wrong for being what it is, I'll have no power (no effectiveness) in the matter.

In this point of view, the game would be to see what that part of me is incomplete about – what that part of me has been unable to express. And while thinking about that, I caught a flash that it could be self-loathing about something.

So I'm looking at granting "being" to some sad or angry or disapproving part of me, acknowledging it, being in compassionate acceptance for the pain or fear that is incomplete in it. I'll let it get complete.

Mind you, I'm not saying I intend to have a warm fuzzy-lovey relationship with self-destruction. :) But I have a friend who overcame an unbeatable case of hepatitis-C, and I remembered that he used an approach similar to this, among other things.

I'm not about to stop doing all the treatments I'm doing. But I'm also getting a strong sense that it makes no sense that I'd have a self-destructive thing growing inside of me.

And as part of that I'll look for an additional name for it, a name that embodies the spirit in which I want to transform this thing. The idea is that if the unexpressed can get complete, a new future and a new world of possibility can become available.

We shall see.

Sunday, February 25, 2007 12:18 AM

Sylvester it is. That's what I'll call the tumor.

When I first read Mom's suggestion in the Guestbook it didn't connect with me. But as I thought about it, it struck me funny: I pictured naughty old Sylvester as the part of me that went goofy and keeps trying nasty mischief. And sweet innocent Tweetie Bird goes wide-eyed and says "Ohhhhhhh, Puddy Tat, I don't tink you sposed to DO dat!" And I started giggling.

97

I couldn't stop: I laughed for ten minutes. And the next thing that hit me was the idea that this whole thing could be viewed as an ongoing comic drama between two cartoon characters.

And I get to think of myself as Tweetie. :-)

It's so perfect, too: as Lindsey's mom and I were raising her as a little kid, when Lindsey made a mistake of any size, Lindsey would hear something like "Oops, you didn't mean to do that, DID you!" And she'd get to try again. That kind of compassion, understanding, forgiveness is a great thing to visualize for the world.

It's a little weird to apply that to Sylvester, but it fits well in my gloriously mixed-up view of the world! All that matters to me is that any part of me that "went Sylvester" on me can be forgiven and welcomed back to the healthy side of the farce.

Wednesday, March 11, 2009

Extraordinary example of the mind's influence on well-being

A friend writes: "If you ever needed an example of the mind's influence on disease, please take a look at the following graph. Wow." (To read the article, go to http://www.maytal.co.il/englishar.htm and search for "Impact of exposure to war stress".)

The article is about relapses of multiple sclerosis during the Hamas war in Israel in 2006. The caption reads "Number of relapses per month. Eighteen relapses occurred during the 33 days of the war compared with one to six relapses in comparable time periods over the 12 months preceding the war. There was no increase in relapse rates during the 3 months that followed the war compared with the same period of the previous year."

Brings to mind a couple of thoughts:

It strongly reminds me that during my own illness, I put a high priority on the power of my state of mind. At all times, even when all the information was not encouraging, instead of pondering all that for no benefit, I asked myself (and often said in my online journal), "Why fill the mind with things that won't make a difference?"

Note: as those who read my journal know, I wasn't in denial – I'm talking about where I chose to focus my consciousness.

It reminds me, in a new way, of the sixties poster that said "War is bad for children and other living things."

Sunday, March 22, 2009

Reality is what it is, regardless of what we think

It's come time for me to say publicly something I've been saying since the beginning of my cancer case 26 months ago. It has to do with the power of our attitude, how we choose to view our circumstances.

> Reality is what it is,
> whether we know it or not,
> and regardless of what we think.

In my community of other kidney cancer e-patients on ACOR, people are repeatedly faced with news they never wanted to hear, uncertainty, circumstances they were not raised to deal with. I know what that feels like, and no matter what your circumstances are today, chances are good that you too will face this – for yourself, a parent, a child, a loved family member, a loved friend.

The other day in my ACOR community a woman named Sally (not her real name) wrote wondering about the decisions she and her husband are facing along the way. Here's my response.

◆   ◆   ◆

Sally, I feel for you. I well remember those days in my case, knowing that what we had to do was educate ourselves and assess our choices. There was no way to know how it was going to turn out. It felt desperate at times. I'll never forget reading those words on the web pages for my disease: "Outlook is bleak." "Prognosis is grim."

I think everyone deals with this differently. After the initial shock I found myself saying "reality is what it is, whether we know it or not. I had cancer before the diagnosis; I have cancer after the diagnosis. The main difference is that now I know it. This is scary, but it also means I have much better ability to deal with it. What are my choices?"

With that approach, I had the experience that knowing I have cancer is empowering and enabling, MUCH better than not realizing it.

(I should note that for years I've taken courses from Landmark Education, a personal growth company that among other things teaches us to be clear about the difference between how things are and our thoughts about them.) As I say, everyone's different. I personally have a strong gut feel that attitude makes a big difference, and the relatively new field of psycho-neuro-immunology supports this: they're studying how mood/attitude (psych) affects the nervous system (neuro) which ties to the immune system. There's real evidence now that attitude can boost the immune system. So I want my attitude to be strong, action-oriented, rather than victim-oriented.

Some might rightly say I'm a "victim" of cancer but for me there's no use in that.

We know that thousands of years ago the function of our anxiety was to help us be alert when a tiger might be about to pounce, so we could take action. Today, when we learn we have cancer, we get anxious and we take action. Beyond that moment, the anxiety has outlived its usefulness. So sometimes I'd remind myself "Yes, this stinks. Thank you for the alarm, Mr. Anxiety. Now, what are my options?"

All the while, I knew these really might be my end days. But there was no use for any other attitude than "what are my options?" With the attitude I chose, I became better able to fully experience life if it DID turn out to be my end days.

I also found that being in touch with my community (family, online CaringBridge journal, etc.) about my status, thoughts, and feelings would help clear my mind. From them, I got back messages of support and encouragement. And some of them said "I can't believe you're being this way about it. You're amazing." And that left me feeling "Huh, maybe I can beat this thing, regardless of the odds."

♦   ♦   ♦

Think about this, too: none of us knows how long we'll live, and patients with a fatal diagnosis have (oddly enough) the advantage of knowing that it's time to wake up and pay attention now. No sudden death for us, nosirree; we have advance notice.

My advice to patients everywhere, regardless of circumstance: Use your mind as an asset, not a liability.

No matter where you are in your journey, choose to be present in the moment, clear about your choices, and the master of your attitude.

Or, as my wonderful sister says about the game of life:

"Must be present to win."

♦   ♦   ♦

Friday, April 13, 2007 5:13 PM

[During the week-long pause in 1st Interleukin treatment]

My relationship to my cancer

Wednesday night I had an enormous realization about my relationship to this cancer. It's unfolding in an unexpected way. I imagine I'll have more to say later, but at this moment I'm willing to say this:

1. I had a conversation with a Landmark friend about severe episodes of retching I'd been having, which would last 15-20 minutes, producing nothing. They disrupted sleep and certainly disrupted my peace of mind and sense of well-being.

2. Shortly after the call with my friend, I had the worst-ever episode.

3. I then settled into bed and had the experience of curling up in a healing cocoon of white energy.

4. The retching has not returned.

I know enough about cause & effect, rationality, and science to know that sequence doesn't prove causation. And I know that the treatment itself has its course, as I just described before. But if you have any interest at all in my personal experience of having cancer, then please hear this: in that call I saw something about my relationship to the cancer and something has shifted.

I won't make any medical predictions and I don't mind whether anyone finds this plausible – but this is my blog and I'm sayin' what I want. :) That's what blogs are for. And I say, this has to do with who I choose to be, in the face of the fact that there's cancer in my life.

(Sorry if that doesn't make sense yet – I'll do what I can to clarify it as time goes by.)

More on this later, as there's more to say.

Be good to each other.

Sunday, April 15, 2007 11:44 PM

Week 2 approaches

This Tuesday I'll start my second week of Interleukin-2. What's so is that I'm not particularly happy about it. It's not a joy ride physically, but more importantly to me, a few weeks from now, we'll learn whether the whole Interleukin-2 process is working for me, or not.

So, ladies and gents, this week I start down a path that leads directly to one of many forks in the cancer road. And this confronts me just a little bit with the mortality and uncertainty of it all.

Having realized that, what to do? I choose to say "Yeah, no kidding, one of those turning points is approaching. Not fun, eh?" And I reconnect with what I chose in the first place: know what my options are, choose my path, and move forward.

Being at peace with it all – even the abyss

This part won't be fun for some of you. It wasn't for me.

Last night, in the middle of the night, I found myself unable to be with the worst possible outcome – that all treatments fail and I die, leaving my family and all of you behind. (Obviously that's not the outcome I'm creating –   but I find that I have no power over anything that I can't squarely imagine. So when I notice I can't be with something, it's time to get to work, or risk the peril of an unknowable challenge.)

Ginny and I talked about it for about an hour. (In bed, lights out, 3 in the morning. That's partnership.) She said that she'd had to face that contingency months ago, and that left her with the freedom to act freely with each day's reality. The problem for me, of course, is different from everyone else's. MY problem is that if I go Lights Out, I simultaneously say goodbye to every single person and everything I love in my life.

We cried a bit, I let go of trying to control everything, and let myself just face the abyss of an uncontrollable future. I let myself see "Yeah, that really might happen. Crap." And when we fell asleep again, I slept deeply and richly. And in the morning we spent as much time as we wanted, lying in bed and being in bed together, enjoying every moment.

Sunday, April 15, 2007 11:44 PM

Do you have cancer, or does it have you?

If this question's new to you, think about it. When I first got the diagnosis, the cancer sure had me: I was at its mercy. Every change in my outlook came from outside me: it was something that seemed to happen to me, something over which I had no control.

I have a mental image for "the cancer has me." In that image, the cancer is like a big dog with a chew toy (me) in its jaws, shaking the daylights out of it and tossing it around.

The pivotal change came when I chose to get in action and do whatever I could, learn whatever I could. Mind you, who am I to know how to fight a cancer?? Do I know anything about the biology of cancer? No. But now my outlook is that I have a cancer in my life, and I'm doing what I can to manage it .... and I'm creating new ways to interact with it, beyond what others have thought of. (Your feedback here tells me that.)

I say it's vitally important that YOU realize what a difference this makes. Remember something I said back in February: citing a study, a nurse in my email group said, "If you're actively involved in creating your care, learning everything you can, and finding the best care available, then your outcome automatically moves to above the median."

Sunday, April 22, 2007 9:27 AM

[During 1st round of Interleukin, 2nd week of treatment]

Guided imagery CD

I know many of you are well into mind-body topics but I want to share this with everyone.

Ginny found a CD titled "Self-Healing with Guided Imagery," by Andrew Weil and Martin Rossman. Disc one is teaching/lecture, and disc two is an excellent recording of three imagery exercises.

The exercises are very similar to some recordings I listened to 25 years ago when I was first interested in mind-body things.

The publisher is Sounds True, www.SoundsTrue.com, but their CDs are often displayed on kiosks in the whole foods section of grocery stores, at least here in the Boston area.

Monday, April 30, 2007 6:02 PM

Renewing connections

A wonderful thing about the last three months, often surprising me, is how many people I've reconnected with – people from years ago. In the past 2 weeks three in particular from college years have come along: Steve Owades, Mark Fishman and Doug

104

White. I had a terrific visit from Steve in the hospital, had the best conversation of my life with Mark, and on Saturday I surprised Doug at his birthday dinner with his family.

I must say that it was a LOT of fun to go scootering through an upscale seafood restaurant and abruptly appear at Doug's table (behind a wall) and say "Hello!" His eyes truly popped wide open. I have a feeling that the idea of a deBronkart appearing out of nowhere, on a scooter no less, was about as probable as Zaphod Beeblebrox appearing, straight out of *Hitchhiker's Guide to the Galaxy.*

(Come to think of it, that may not be a coincidence.)

But in my view, part of our job in life is to give our friends little surprise moments of brain-jolt, little bursts of neurochemicals that they never expected. Keeps 'em nimble.

Tuesday, May 8, 2007 8:32 PM

You'll recall the Andrew Weil CD that I mentioned. The visualization exercise talks about imagining a safe place, and for some reason I got that for me it's the ocean, listening to waves at night. That reminded both Ginny and me that when we were college age, decades before we met, we both liked "The Sea," an album of Rod McKuen's poems intermixed with background music and ocean sounds. Some years back I bought Ginny the CD version of The Sea, so we got it out and we've been playing it after lights out. It takes us both back to a time of wonderful futures, and that's a great place to be. (I never get to hear the end of the album..... zzzzzz.)

Saturday, May 12, 2007 11:07 AM

Amazing music news

This happened Wednesday but I couldn't quite believe it so I didn't post it until now. It's about my chorus's annual show, a week from tonight. I'm going to be on stage, singing! This is totally unexpected. (Heck, I only know half the repertoire.)

Here's what happened. Wednesday at chorus rehearsal I was, as usual, sitting on my scooter observing. When a song came along that I love, I'd perform it with joy. (Barbershop singing isn't just about singing: expression/performance is judged, too.) After repeated gestures from the risers (and knowing it's okay with the director), I slowly inched my scooter up to the end of the risers, as I've done at some recent rehearsals.

Then at break time, our performance coach (who teaches the performance category at judging school) came up to me and said, "I want you on stage for the show. You're performing with plenty of passion. For the songs you know, you can pull your scooter on stage. The stage will be set as a piano bar, with some cocktail tables, and you can be a patron. Just pull up to a table. For the songs you don't know, you can pull off stage."

Sooooo, I'm gonna be on stage again, in a most unexpected way. Wow. NOT what I was anticipating a month or two back!

We create a world with how we view life

Now, here's the thing: look how the mental attitude feeds on its own results.

If I'd been doing the "sensible and reasonable" thing for these past few months, acting like you'd expect for someone with a "median survival time 5-1/2 months" cancer, I certainly wouldn't have been out there mentally creating "being healthy," actively enjoying life, getting a scooter and a shiny red car to tote it in (cheaper than the previous car). So I wouldn't have been able to take myself to rehearsal (after a full day of work no less), and might not have been energetic enough to be joyfully performing like that.

But I did what I did, and now I'm going to be on stage.

Of course, the treatment that we choose (and vigorously pursue) is a huge part of it. But a person could be totally asleep and receive treatments. How we are in our minds, especially what we create in our interpretation of our human experience, makes a

106

vast difference. Don't ever forget that. And the support you give me continues to be a big contribution.

Several times my chorus has sung "You'll never walk alone" for me.

As fellow cancer blogger Leroy Sievers wrote: "Obviously, I'm not bashful about talking about cancer. It's a little too late for that. As I continue to do this, it becomes easier. It's a conversation with friends. And all of you bring up ideas that I had never thought of.

"But I do have an answer to the question, 'What do you get out of writing the blog?': A daily reminder that none of us walks this road alone. What could be better than that?"

Being on stage for the annual show. THAT's what could be better than that!

Sunday, May 13, 2007 9:56 AM

The freedom to live now

I'm going to use this spot to reply to a guestbook note from my uncle Jim McCulloh, because I've received related thoughts in emails from others, too.

Jim, yes, being abruptly confronted with our mortality can very much set us free, after a chain of events. You get the terror, the realizations, the information about your odds.... and once it's settled in, people often find themselves feeling more free to be alive than ever.

Usually when I make a generalization like that I'll add "in my experience," but in this case I didn't because I've seen it said over and over in different places. It's part of Dr. Bernie Siegel's "Extraordinary Cancer Patient" materials, and shows up all through cancer blogs. (Leroy Sievers' blog is one example.)

In my view this is because the mortality confrontation makes us give up our focus on "It'll all turn out someday," so we start living NOW.

We all know we'll die, but usually that's "somewhere out there," not in the foreseeable future.

I remember vividly how my view of life changed when I got the news that death was quite literally in the foreseeable future, like maybe within months.

That experience has us drop our thoughts about someday, and start being PRESENT in our lives, living now. We are set free from all the reasons we had NOT to live now.

It shows up in cancer writings all over the place: people say they're taking more joy in every day, every moment.

As many people on this blog know, that's also what you get from the courses given by Landmark Education: you learn to not be run by the many interpretations that we as humans put on our daily experiences.

One result, as the Landmark web site says, is "the freedom to be at ease no matter what the circumstance." Surely that's what I'm experiencing. (I've taken 5 Landmark courses and have been on the teams that work with course leaders to produce the results for others.)

Interestingly, what flows out of that freedom is usually breakthroughs in relationships, even when that's not what people were looking for when they signed up.

Another common result is to have all kinds of unreasonable things start happening – like being invited to be on stage when I only know half the repertoire.

Believe me, we have no IDEA what's possible when we start living authentically in the moment. No idea. So yes, when we get present in the moment, we do get set free: free to be who we always would have authentically been, if nothing had stopped us. And I must say, the one-weekend Landmark courses are a far simpler route than waiting until you get cancer. :-) My Landmark training is what gave me the freedom to be how I've been, through this whole process. Thanks for asking. Good question.

Thursday, May 22, 2008 8:42 PM, EDT

Tonight a friend asked how much of a role I think you (my community) played in my recovery, compared to the medication. Who can tell? What I do know is that emotions and support are well documented as being beneficial to the immune system, and that's a good thing.

Sunday, June 8, 2008 10:40 PM, EDT

The therapeutic value of blogging

The *Scientific American* blog reports:

Blogging–It's Good for You: The therapeutic value of blogging becomes a focus of study

Scientists (and writers) have long known about the therapeutic benefits of writing about personal experiences, thoughts and feelings. But besides serving as a stress-coping mechanism, expressive writing produces many physiological benefits. Research shows that it improves memory and sleep, boosts immune cell activity and reduces viral load in AIDS patients, and even speeds healing after surgery. A study in the February issue of *The Oncologist* reports that cancer patients who engaged in expressive writing just before treatment felt markedly better, mentally and physically, as compared with patients who did not. ...

No surprise to us! Thanks to E-Patient Scholar Susannah Fox for this tip.

♦   ♦   ♦

We left off our storyline in May 2007, just as I was about to go on stage for my chorus's annual show. Well, you know what they say to performers before they go on stage ...

Chapter 10: "Break a Leg"

May 15 - June 17, 2007

"He got up to go to bathroom; I heard him say 'I don't feel so good,' then he fell. He was rolled in a ball, unconscious. ....I knew the leg was broken and why."

– Ginny

On Monday, May 14, I had the scheduled CT scan. It would prove to be my last with the iodine dye that they sometimes use to enhance contrast, because at 5:30 the next morning I had a not-uncommon side effect: I fainted – with a significant consequence.

Tuesday, May 15, 2007 1:16 PM

Hi all, Ginny here.

Today the writing will not be so eloquent. Dave got up to use the facilities at 5:30 this a.m. and fainted. He fell and landed on his left leg...the one with the metastasis. It broke as was predicted it might.

We had an emergency plan in place and it worked well. The ambulance came and transported him to our local ER; got some pain medicine and a traction splint and sent him to Beth Israel Deaconess Hosp. If his oncologist gives the OK, he'll be in surgery tomorrow. The orthopedic surgeon and assoc. stopped by. Tentative plan is to put an intermedullary pin down through the middle of the bone and a plate on the outside of the bone and bone cement to fill in the gaps.

For those of a medical background, it was a steep oblique fracture of the distal femur. When I saw the picture at the ER, it didn't look very displaced. He had a traction splint on within 1/2 hour of the fracture. His blood pressure was very low causing the fall.

The docs are going to come in and put in a nerve block so the leg will stop spasming until we can get him to surgery. I guess they do that a lot on the battlefield to transport soldiers when they have injuries.

All in all, we are both hanging in there. I'll let you know when something new comes up. Ginny

Tuesday, May 15, 2007 5:06 PM

Hi, just a footnote. Dave's oncologist hasn't visited us yet, but has moved us to the oncology ward where treatment is VERY special. We are now in Stoneman 746, the same room we started Interleukin treatment in!

Dave is feeling comfortable. Thanks for all the prayers today (and everyday). Ginny

Wednesday, May 16, 2007 6:44 AM

Hi, it's Dave back again.

I'm just amazed at how rapidly things are moving. I may be taking my first steps without a walker TONIGHT!

Today I'll have the surgery to repair the femur.

As planned, Dr. Megan Anderson will clean out the area where the cancer did its dirty work. She'll fill the resulting space with bone cement. She'll then insert a steel pin running the length of the bone, and add a steel plate on the outside – a "belt and suspenders" combination that will be extra strong.

She says typically such patients are released to go home just three to four days after surgery. That would be this weekend!

And, get this: I'm allowed to use the leg (put my weight on it) IMMEDIATELY, as soon as the anesthesia wears off. Like, today.

Hard to believe.

Mind you, I may take steps today, but I won't be fully back to normal for a while. The leg's muscles have atrophied in these 10 weeks, and Dr. Anderson said it takes longer to regain the strength than the length of the atrophy. (In other words it may be 3 months before I'm truly walking around as if nothing happened.)

To support that, before I'm released they'll assess my strength and coordination. They may refer me to a rehab place to strengthen my walking muscles, or maybe just have the physical therapist visit at home a few more times.

Ginny feels confident I won't need to go to rehab.

♦   ♦   ♦

Take responsibility for yourself

If you're ever hospitalized (or have any complex care), never forget that you need to understand what they're doing and why. Do not assume everyone knows everything important about you. Be vigilant; think ahead.

Here are some examples from my own treatment:

- To be sure I could tolerate Interleukin I needed qualifying tests – a routine stress test and pulmonary function test. When they tried to schedule me for the usual treadmill stress test I pointed out that it wouldn't work, given my lame leg, and they said "Good catch!" Instead, they gave me a 4-hour non-exercise stress test.

- Before my surgery they sent a letter about preparation. It said to get a bottle of magnesium citrate and drink it the day before. Well, that's a laxative that really cleans you out. So I asked "With this leg, I won't want to be running to the office rest room, will I?" "Good point," they said. "You better plan to work from home that day."

- We were treating the leg, hoping it might get better, but we knew there was a chance the leg would eventually break. I was sure they had a plan for what we'd do if that happened, so I asked, and it turns out that with everything else going on, there was no plan yet. So we made one up, on the spot. And as you've just seen, that made a big difference when the time came.

If you want to know more – a lot more – about this kind of "medical self-defense" thinking, read Trisha Torrey's excellent book *You Bet Your Life: Ten Mistakes Every Patient Makes*. We might like to think that each of us has our own private NASA, with everything all thought out – but even NASA makes fatal mistakes sometimes.

Healthcare is complex. Do your part to help think things out. You've got enough drama as it is – help prevent more.

Any entrepreneurs out there? I bet there would be a big market for a supercharged suspension for ambulances. The ambulance that drove me to Boston yesterday sure didn't have one – every bump in the hour-long trip sent my thigh muscles into spasm. I got to be pretty good at doing Lamaze-style breathing and puffing, and the EMT kept an eye out the windshield to tell me when one was coming. It helped.

◆   ◆   ◆

Meanwhile, good news on the Interleukin front. The CAT scans did indeed get done yesterday. The tumor board hasn't done their full assessment yet (we'll get their "verdict" next Monday), but my oncologist Dr. McDermott says the two biggest mets in the lungs have shrunk!

A smaller lung met grew some, but if I understand correctly, the essential news is that there HAS been a response to the IL-2. That means I'm in the lucky group that does get a response! So I anticipate getting a Yes to proceed with more of it this summer.

But first, there will be another set of scans four weeks from now. (You may recall that immunotherapy keeps working over an extended period of time.)

That's all for now – more news as it happens!

Thursday, May 17, 2007 8:38 AM

The surgery went great! I have very little discomfort and I'll be out of bed today. (I did not stand on the leg last night; will probably do so today.)

All the docs who've seen me today say I look great. (I always love it when someone tells me that.)

Friday will be a "grueling day of physical therapy" as the PTs work to get me in good walking condition, awakening the muscles in the bad leg.

btw, I continue to be very moved by the wonderful things you say, in the guestbook, in emails, and in cards. It makes SUCH a difference to know I'm cared for. Thanks.

Friday, May 18, 2007 9:25 AM

Thursday I did succeed in getting out of bed, as planned. I stood, unassisted but shaky, for a few seconds, then got into a recliner. I spent a couple of hours being comfortable there.

In bed I started doing the recommended exercises, and started flexing the knee, to bring it to the standard "sit in bed with your knees raised" position. That was NOT comfortable, partly because of sore muscles and partly because of the gigantic Ace bandage that was wrapped around my thigh to control swelling.

This morning the surgeon removed the Ace bandage. I showed her my knee flex and her face lit up. She said some people don't get to that point for two months.

That's all for now. Wish me luck today with the "grueling" PT sessions – they say I'll spend a half hour actually walking, today, first with a walker and then maybe without.

Love,

Dave

Friday, May 18, 2007 10:38 PM

Friday actually turned out to be a fairly annoying and frustrating day.

I was so eager to make as much progress as possible on walking. I had a good visit with a PT, who set up a walker and took me on my first foray out of the room and down the hall. It went well. Later an Occupational Therapist (OT) talked about the geography of my workplace and home, and did some preliminary leg lifting with me, which immediately led to an improvement in my leg's range of motion and ability to lift the leg off the floor. (Painful, but not unbearable.)

As you might imagine, I was eager for more of that! I asked the OT, and he said he'd try to arrange for some co-op students to come assist me. I thought he meant "this afternoon."

But it turns out that you get one PT visit per day, no matter what the situation. If you're in a rehab hospital you get as much as you want.

Mind you, this is a one-time upset: now that I know the rules, I know what to expect and how to deal with it. But it's ANNOYING to my impatience department.

Somebody else said, in passing, "You can have a nurse do some of these exercises with you." But I didn't ask for that, because I thought more PTs were coming.

Anyway, tonight I had a good conversation to complete all this, with a nurse I'd never met before, who deserves a prize for listening skills. She also convinced me that it's not dangerous to use pain meds when doing the leg stretches.

This afternoon I had another good visit from classmate Stephen Owades, and last night Sandy and Lindsey came over after work. When I'm in for an Interleukin treatment guests aren't that easy, but this is a routine hospitalization, and guests are easy and good to have.

Saturday, May 19, 2007 5:10 PM

Today I stood on both legs, unassisted, for the first time since February. WOOHOO!

And there's a chance I'll be going home tomorrow (Sunday). Not definite, but a chance.

This was a big shift, after Friday's frustrations. I could have stayed frustrated but I looked more deeply into what was upsetting for me, and had conversations with several staff people that got to the bottom of things, and got everything clear. What became possible, then, was effective communication. Amazing!

And today I had conversations, starting with the 6:30am doctor visit, including a 3pm comment from an MD that there's a good chance I'll go home Sunday. Wow!

So this evening and Sunday we're working on weaning me off the IV pain med, and ensuring that I can sit up, stand up, walk, and sit down as well as I could before the Tuesday accident. When that criterion is met, I'll be safe to send home.

EV'BODY SAY YEAH!! Thank you!

Sunday, May 20, 2007 6:22 PM

Today's post is, to me, sobering but ultimately uplifting.

Bottom line is that I'm still in the hospital and glad to be here, because my leg is very swollen and it hurts.

There was a big factor at play, the past couple of days, that I knew about but didn't comprehend. (I may get some details wrong.)

When I went into surgery, they inserted something at the top of my leg called a nerve block. I have the impression that this is fairly new for my kind of case; it's being used in Iraq for the initial treatment for wound victims, to reduce pain during transport, instead of morphine. (All the staff who were talking about it here were impressed with its many benefits.)

The nerve block line stayed in through the surgery and through last night. It's a drip, through a catheter, but it's not IV .... it delivers the anesthetic into a general area where the nerve (or bundle of nerves) starts. The nerves soak in a sort-of puddle of this stuff.

The nerve block worked marvelously on me. (As brother Ken said today, "I gotcha – you're having the pain, you just don't know it.") I would have happily kept it in for a long time, except for two limitations:

1. I can't go home hooked to a dripping catheter.

2. It not only blocks pain nerves, it blocks strength nerves. Soooo, the better the pain relief, the more useless the leg. :-)

So on Saturday, wanting to go home, I was motivated to remove the thing. We reduced its setting from 15 to 10, then to 5, each time taking those walks that I described, to see how the strength returned. Everything did go exactly as well as I described yesterday.

116

But there was one thing Dr. Anderson, the bone surgeon, told me that didn't sink in at first, as she marveled at my results: "You may have completely skipped the whole first two days [of pain], and they're the worst. They can be excruciating." Since I was feeling fine Saturday evening, I figured I'd dodged the bullet without knowing it.

But it took longer for the remaining "puddle" to clear from my system, and today I found out what the tail-end of the pain curve feels like. So did my thigh: it was already swollen but the swelling increased till the thigh looked like a huge bratwurst, which didn't really like bending at the knee.

I did take a couple of test walks. My strength is good, my gait is good, but the pain prevents me from going far.

All of this is sobering when I think of the pain I might have experienced this week, and didn't.

But it's also uplifting when I realize the continuing work that medical people are doing, to find new treatments (like nerve blocks) or new applications (like using them for early wound treatment). To me this is one of the prime reasons to choose one of the major teaching hospitals: it's where folks are most likely to know about the new stuff.

Strengthwise I'm in good enough shape to go back to work, but I don't know how long it'll take for the swelling and pain to clear up. Soooo, once again, friends & family, I find myself saying: "We'll see how tomorrow goes"!

p.s. If you want a sobering thought, consider how things went here today for the nurses and docs whom I was grilling as I sought to understand what the heck was happening! (I was nice, but believe me, I was focused and intentional in my questions....)

Monday, May 21, 2007 11:39 AM

I'm headed home!

It's hard to understand how rapidly things are moving. Yesterday was so swollen and painful. Today the leg is still swollen but the pain's much less and the leg strength is surprisingly good.

The first few doctors I saw today all said their view of things looked great, so as far as they're concerned I can go home. So I've been up and about in my room, using my walker – spent about an hour getting things done, on my feet: Gave myself a spongebath at the sink, started gathering possessions, clearing out accumulated clutter.

Ah, Dr. McDermott (who "owns" me except for the bones) just came by and gave the final word: we can go!

I'll see ya when we're back in the 603 area code.

Dave

Monday, May 21, 2007 9:11 PM

Y'all, we are home (for several hours), having stopped for several must-do-today errands. Very tired, good to be home in bed.

Thanks to those who've volunteered to Davey-sit already, on Wednesday and Thursday!

A new physical therapist will visit Tuesday. The PT and I have a lot of work to do on this leg, to get it back to where it was. The time's not set yet, so I don't know when/if I'll have an opening for company.

p.s. Ginny is a martyr, except not really, because she doesn't do the "woe is me" part or the "killing myself" part. She's just an incredibly generous and loving contributor, even when she herself is exhausted.

Tuesday, May 22, 2007 2:20 PM

Cripes, I'm nearly walking already. What is UP with this?

I'm sure it'll be some weeks before I'm allowed to discard my walker, and return the scooter to its rental home, but I can now stand in the middle of my walker and basically .... walk! Without leaning on it. To the contrary, I'm basically pushing it along in front of me.

Recovery status: walking doesn't give me leg or joint pain, but I do have 20 pounds of swelling in that leg, and THAT hurts when I stand for long. We're managing it with medication, but it still hurts. Anyway, I guess I got no excuse now: I can't say "Gotta be careful, I might break my leg" because I already did so! And the result is two perfectly good legs.

.... heh heh heh.... I just had an awfully bratty thought.... my chorus sings "You'll Never Walk Alone" for me, but have I got news for THEM! HA!

Thursday, May 24, 2007 10:40 AM

Update: "Activities of Daily Living" (aka ADL)

ADL is the big buzzword in rehab – your ability to handle normal daily activities: getting dressed, showering, going to work, etc.

Being able to stand on the left leg has given me a big breakthrough in ADL. It means I can do all sorts of useful things:

- step into the shower, without sitting on a pivoting barstool
- walk up a step! (It was a tiny one but I did it!) (With walker)
- step out of my pants while standing. (This is more of a big deal than you might think ... consider standing in the bathroom, held up by a walker, without putting weight on the left leg, and trying to remove your trousers! Now I can do it, no problem.)

Perhaps most important (to me) is that since I can put weight on both legs, I no longer need the platform walker! I removed the [ugly!!!] platform attachment, and just use it as a regular rolling walker. This lets me practice my regular walking gait for the first time in months.

Busy Day

Had a VERY busy/active day Wednesday.

In the morning, my very good barbershop singer buddy Matt visited. We went for a drive, with me driving. It felt like being a teenager again – we were just cruisin' in the car, looking for what's next. It felt like freedom.

The high point was our stop at Dunkin Donuts – for weeks I've had a mild craving for glazed donuts. I had two, and an iced coffee – my first coffee since January!

My afternoon buddy was George, a guy I worked with way back at the start of my career. He was a visionary manager, pulling together a group of unknowns in the company. He made us superstars.

Most of us, including him, were born the same year – we were 27 at the time.

How often do you see a manager (his first mgmt job) who can pull off something like that? I've never seen anything like it since. And it wasn't a flash in the pan; he went on to be very successful in top-level positions in several companies.

And then, I went to chorus rehearsal – the whole 3-1/2 hours. I sang some and surprised a lot of people – they'd hoped to have me on stage for last weekend's annual show, but then the broken leg happened. So it was a real surprise to see me already, especially with no cast!

That was a busy day, and I am TIRED this morning. I think I shall nap after the physical therapist finishes.

Anniversary weekend

Seven years ago this weekend Ginny and I stood on the front steps of our house and recited our home-made vows, formalizing this marriage. Two weeks later we went on a business trip to Paris, aka "Woohoo, free honeymoon in Paris!" It was a splendid start to what has been a splendid marriage. I cannot believe the love and generosity I receive every day from this wonderful woman.

Friday, May 25, 2007 10:04 PM

Well, boys and girls, today is the start of our anniversary weekend, and I'm going to summarize all the treatment results so far, because the news is quite good! I got an email from the surgeon Friday, with the lab results from last week's bone surgery. One part of the surgery was to remove any tumor cells (dead or alive) in the femur before filling the hole with cement. The removed cells were sent to the lab, because we want to know if the leg tumor responded to the radiation we gave it before the kidney came out. So we've been waiting to see the lab report from the surgery. We combined that with the scan results Dr. McDermott gave us from the scan 5/17, and here's how it adds up:

Kidney (the primary tumor) and adrenal gland:

• Entire organs removed – tumors are gone.

Lung mets (treated with Interleukin):

• The 2 biggest shrank substantially

• 1 is unchanged

• The 2 smallest grew some

Femur (treated with radiation in March):

• The cells she scraped out were mostly dead (that is, the tumor did respond to the radiation)

• Other parts of the femur showed no additional tumor (good news)

Skull (I had one tiny met just inside the forehead; it was treated with Interleukin):

• Gone.

Left ulna: (treated only by Interleukin):

• No improvement yet. (Radiation is coming up.)

Right thigh (a 1″ met inside the muscle):

• Results unknown – it wasn't covered in these scans

This means the entire remaining "tumor load" is

- The 2 larger lung mets, reduced
- The 3 smaller lung mets
- The forearm (radiation hasn't started yet)
- The right thigh (1" intramuscular)

I think this is a FINE way to start the summer. PAARRRTY!!!! Love, Dave & Ginny

p.s. Thanks for your support and the results you've been causing!

Monday, May 28, 2007 10:25 PM

Quick update – it's been a great holiday weekend here in the Boston area.

My leg strength continues to improve. Whenever possible, I no longer use the aluminum/geriatric-looking walker; I'm back to using the wonderful Hugo Rolling Walker from www. HugoAnywhere.com. Great company. The Hugo has hand brakes, a box to carry things in, and a seat to either rest on or carry other things on top of. (Until you've been tied to a walker, you have no idea how useful these tote options are.) Hugo products are 1,000% ahead of everything else in the business.

Mind you, this item isn't appropriate for everything – it requires that I either stoop way over or stand straight up and just push it along in front. But for my stage of recuperation it's perfect. I took a few steps this weekend completely unassisted. I'm nowhere near to being completely free of gadgets but we're progressing there rapidly. I'm hoping to return to the office (again) this week but the physical therapy people aren't so sure I'm ready. So the office is lining up some tasks that can be done from home or office. That's enough for now.

Emerging from months of having our priorities elsewhere, we're rediscovering the world of bill payment, selling that MN house, etc. Keep them cards 'n' letters comin' in, because they REALLY make a difference. We may be in a time of few symptoms, but I still have cancer cells in this bod, so there's still work to do! Love, Dave & Ginny

Wednesday, May 30, 2007 6:48 AM

I just want to say that it makes SUCH a difference to have two working legs, even if they're not 100%. (My left leg is usually still wobbly – I don't have full strength back, yet.)

I can get out of the car now and, if necessary, hang onto the top of the car (there's a finger-grippable ridge there) as I walk past the back door, or walk to the trunk. This makes all the difference compared to my previous need to haul the walker out of the front seat, even if I only wanted to go to the back of the car.

One of my major skills of recent months was what they call "transfers" – moving my butt from one seat to another, e.g. from wheelchair to bed or toilet. Now I'm reverting to just plain old "stand up, sit down."

The left leg still swells – standard post-surgical swelling. It's less than before but it's improving on schedule. And it responds well to the Comprilan "low stretch" elastic bandages that sister Amy told me about. She's a physical therapist who works a lot with edema (swelling). She said low-stretch bandages are much better than Ace bandages for edema because low stretch works with the muscles to pump excess fluid back to where it belongs.

Meanwhile, with the doctor's okay, last night Ginny removed the staples from my incisions on the left leg – a small milestone on the road to recovery.

Time for work now, and chorus tonight. Have hundreds of good days today, all you hundreds of supporters out there!

Friday, June 1, 2007 4:06 PM

COULD IT BE? Yes it could.... It appears that we have a buyer for our Minnesota house!

I already have a palpable sense of relief, as our load is lightened.

When that deal closes, we'll no longer be dragging the past around – we'll only need to work on the present and what we can see of the future. MUCH better!

Dave

Sunday, June 3, 2007 10:37 AM

It's been a great week. Yesterday we went to the Red Sox - Yankees game, which was a huge treat, made even better by the 11-6 victory we inflicted on The Evil Ones. (Hey, a rivalry is a rivalry.) Our wheelchair-accessible seats had superb visibility, and they were on the top row of the section (of course), which means they were also right near the food windows and rest rooms. Daughter Lindsey and beau Jon had seats in the next section over. We got there early enough to indulge in the street vendors, buying shirts and sausage. All in all it was an entirely satisfying day.

I was surprised at how the wheelchair made it easier to get around at Fenway Park. The crowd at a Sox game (or Patriots game, for that matter) is usually a bunch of grunting bulls, but they parted graciously for me wherever I went. (It was easier to send me for food than for Ginny to go get it.)

This was also the week where I returned to work post-fracture, and the week where we got our deal on selling the house. Wow. Speaking of which, here's something that the rational among us are just going to have to shut up and deal with. Have you heard of the thing about burying a statue of St. Joseph upside down, to speed up the sale of a house?

This weekend I learned from sister Suede that, unbeknownst to me, a college friend of hers DID go onto my property, in the dark of night, black clothes and all, and bury the statue according to the legend. And they did this a week before my buyer showed up. Yes, boys and girls, make of it whatever you want. I'm anything but superstitious. All I know is, after a year, I have an agreement on my house. (I don't have a closed sale yet! But I do have an agreement.)

124

What's your "drop dead date"?

Next weekend is my college class's 35th reunion. This past February (when my outlook was highly uncertain) there were quite a few classmates taking a stand that I would be at the reunion, despite the medical statistics about my "median survival time." Fortunately while in that same college, I learned enough about statistics to see through these stats and not be misled by the first impression.

That statistic I found said the median survival time for a case like mine is 5-1/2 months from the time of diagnosis. My cancer was discovered on January 11. 5.5 months after that is June 26. So I've taken to referring to June 26 as my Drop Dead Date, and I anticipate gleefully thumbing my nose at that date, spraying a big wet razzberry at it as I zoom past. Thank you for all your support through these months. It ain't over yet but I have clear memories of experiencing your support as I lay in my bed, many many days and nights. And now, together we can say, big fat razzberries to the Drop Dead Date!

Sunday, June 3, 2007 8:02 PM

Okay, another two-posting day. (This morning's post is above.)

Yesterday I felt so good after bopping around Fenway Park that today I tried some more things.

After a few tentative steps this afternoon, I walked from one end of the house to the other and back, unassisted. Twice.

Then we went to visit Ginny's daughter Heather. I negotiated the stairs in and out of her apartment building, using nothing but handrail and cane for support. HA!

Rumor says Steven Tyler may be retiring as lead singer of Aerosmith. Somebody please let 'em know – I know a singer who's newly available to go around hollering "Walk this way!" With copious attitude.

Monday, June 4, 2007 10:29 PM

Quoth the doctor: "Dude, slow down!"

Well, that's not quite what she said. But she did say to quit walking around unassisted, i.e. to keep using the walker, so the fractured femur (remember the fracture? it's still in there) can heal some more before we start jumping on pogo sticks again.

Mind you, she and all 4 of her team were all grins, seeing how well things had progressed; and there was much laughter and happiness, recalling that wacky night of surgery, just 19 days ago (!). One doc got to be the Human Traction Machine, hauling on my foot for a few hours, or something like that – don't quote me.

Anyway for now I'm only allowed to put 50% of my weight on that leg, not more. Thpppt.

[Hey... I wonder where she got the news that I've been walking around unassisted! Perhaps they sneak a peek in my journal now and then?? Have we entered a new era in patient-physician communication?]

Dave

p.s. to Mom: Okay, okay, okay – you're vindicated – I know you said I shouldn't rush things. You Were Right.

Thursday, June 7, 2007 10:59 AM

Something's up, inside the leg.

Yesterday at work, while doing my usual walker-walking, I felt a rattly popping sort of thing in the vicinity of the knee. No pain, no big "snap," just "Hm, where did THAT come from?"

It got a bit worse, so today I'm going to see the bone doctor and see what's up. Obviously, I hope this won't interfere with my big college reunion this weekend! But priorities are priorities.

The leg's definitely got something going on. Along the incision there's a stiff area more than an inch wide, and there's some swelling all around, and if I do apply a little pressure to the leg (e.g. while standing), it lets me know this is not a good thing. So something's gone backwards since Tuesday.

This strikes me as a Roseann Roseanna Danna moment: "It's just like my father used to say: It's always something. You kick cancer's ass, and then you get some stupid thing in your leg."

Ah well: remember the lessons – grant it being, don't pretend it's not there, and do what your doctor says. (And your mother.)

Dave

p.s. I forgot to share with you that within the past week the ulna met shrank by at least 50%. The sudden progress raised all our eyebrows, including the bone doc's.

I guess they're not kidding when they say immune therapy (like Interleukin) is long-acting.

Thursday, June 7, 2007 5:10 PM

Quick update to Dave's story. He broke two screws in his bone plate and is currently in surgery again. A friend took him to his Doc. appt. in Boston and she said I can do it this PM so she is doing it NOW!

Will let you all know when I know anything more. No MIT this weekend I guess.

Ginny

Friday, June 8, 2007 2:29 AM

I'm writing this at (holy cow) 2:30 a.m. without my glasses so pardon any typos.

I'm feeling pretty well, pain-wise.

Haven't gotten out of bed yet, nor have I sat up at the bedside. Pain level is as expected; I've got the every-6-minute morphine button. Still hurts, predictably so.

Eager to have lots of visitors drop by from the reunion! So any of y'all who want to come, do.

Friday, June 8, 2007 12:14 PM

I've had my first visit with physical therapy and took my first walk to the loo. All agree that I seem to have some experience with this.

I'll probably be discharged Saturday afternoon, with permission to attend the reunion dinner if I feel up to it. I'll be back in my own bed in N.H. Saturday night. Sunday we'll see.

Next week I can work from home, but no going to the office for now!

Saturday, June 9, 2007 9:41 AM

I've been cleared to be released from the hospital. Now I just need to get some paperwork from them, and produce a certain Output From My Body now that my catheter has been removed. They say I'll probably be outa here mid-afternoon.

REUNION TIME! (Gently.)

Sunday, June 10, 2007 11:31 PM

Hokey smokes, Bullwinkle – I didn't realize it'd been so long since I posted! We did have a great time last night at the reunion dinner. It wasn't just that I got to see people I haven't seen for years – this time I also got to meet people I've known by name but have never met in person, but who greeted me warmly. That's due in large part to this journal. And what a great feeling it was. (I did not dance, despite several invites.)

By the time we got home last night we were both definitely in pain, for real, because this surgery was tougher than last time in several ways, and the rougher my situation is, the more strain there is on Ginny's frame. So this morning we knew we'd want to skip the reunion brunch and games. In fact all we did today was get my new prescriptions filled, get haircuts, and REST.

I'm allowed to work this week but I have to STAY HOME FROM WORK all week, and not argue about it. REST the leg. WEAR THE SPIFFY NEW BRACE whenever upright. Also, this time they used much heftier metal to repair the femur. It seems they're as committed as I am to ensuring that this time it works. Good thing, because I AM GETTING TIRED OF BEING IN THE HOSPITAL and not being at work! (Having said that, I do know that these worries are a heck of a lot better than wondering when I'm going to die. But being a baby boomer, I want it all, thank you.)

Sunday, June 17, 2007 8:47 PM

Here I am once again, having not posted in a week. I've had so much spinning in my head, it's been hard to know where to start. What a week! It's the week since I got out of the hospital after the second leg surgery. During that time I went to the college reunion dinner, spent a week at home mostly resting (physically), got hooked up with a great physical therapist right here in Nashua, went to another reunion dinner with long-ago co-workers, put in a couple of exhilarating days of work from home, had the long-awaited CAT scan for April HDIL-2 results, cleaned my papers and bills out of the dining room for the first time in months, and had a great Father's Day.

Monday I'm returning to work. Mid-afternoon Ginny will fetch me for the long-awaited meeting with the oncology team to assess last week's CAT scans and see what they think is next for my treatment.

Department of transportation

1. Jason the PT is encouraging me to move to crutches. I've always been leery of them (don't want to fall) but I discovered that my fastest walker gait is a "crutch lope," or whatever they call it when a crutchee goes striding along. In other words, I already

know crutchese. Today I used 'em to go to the movies – sure is easier to hoist 'em into a car than any walker!

2. However, for work, I'm reverting to the motorized scooter. Enough of adventurously pushing the limits! The limits bit back, and I don't like it. I want to improve continuously from now on, so I'll use my leg brace and the scooter until the doc & PT change it.

Ulna update

10 days ago I said my ulna met had shrunk by 50%. It's shrunk more! It varies day to day but it's at most the size of a walnut, probably less. My challenge in this situation is to realize that I have 2 different issues in that arm, so I don't get carried away. One issue is the tumor, which may grow or die entirely. But even if it dies, there's still the bone damage: the scallop-shaped scoop that it ate out of the bone. That will repair itself like a fracture, but in the meantime I have to not overload it (with crutch, walker, etc.). My goal is to keep the tumor small and the bone healthy!

De Gustibus Non Est Disputandum

That's Latin for "there's no accountin' fer tastes." Cancer patients commonly report sudden and emphatic changes in their tastes – both their preferences and what foods actually taste like to them. For me the most conspicuous example of this was that I lost all interest in coffee, which is comparable to the Pope losing interest in church.

Well, guess what: in the past few weeks the interest has returned. It's not yet the same as it was months ago, but it's getting stronger both in desire and in taste. Indeed, there's no accountin' for tastes: heaven knows what's actually going on in me, biologically. But here's what it feels like: it feels like my cancer is rewinding entirely, rolling itself back up into wherever it came from. The ulna news fits nicely with that, eh? And together they lead splendidly into this:

HEY, IT'S D D D MINUS 9!

My fictional Drop Dead Date is June 26, and it still doesn't look like I'm headed that way.

I am very in awe of what my community (you, my doctors and caregivers, my supportive co-workers, everyone) have created as an extraordinary experience for my family and me in these months.

Chapter 11: It's official –
I'm a responder!

June 18 – June 26, 2007

Monday, June 18, 2007 8:49 PM

It's official: I am an Interleukin Responder!

I'm in that select minority for whom HDIL-2 (High Dosage Interleukin-2) works. That means my tumors are responding to treatment, and that means I get to have more.

The doctors' report today, evaluating last week's CAT scan, couldn't have been much better:

- The target lesions are "dramatically smaller." They're less than half their previous size.

- My condition is "remarkable" considering where I was three months ago. Dr. McDermott, principal investigator on this Interleuken clinical trial, says, "Back then I wouldn't have bet much money at all on your being where you are now."

In other words, people, WE HAVE KICKED BUTT so far! We have beaten the odds, we have made giant steps toward the goal of Club N.E.D., and the game shall go on!

Next: I qualify for another round – another cycle of "one week in the hospital, one week home, another week in the hospital." It'll probably start a few weeks from now.

I've been telling you it'd be late July or late August, but not so: the clinical trial requires that the next batch start within a certain time. And it turns out there are other rules about (ahem) surgery not muddying the water, medically ... so this broken leg malarkey almost interfered with the much higher priority. Bottom line: the window of opportunity to start round 2 is only a couple of weeks wide!

I propose that this time we set a goal of total victory, leaving the docs SCOURING my innards, looking for traces of a disease that simply ain't there anymore. Waddaya think??

I hope you can imagine how grateful Ginny and I are, for your contributions to my care, your cards, CDs, books, your prayers and other forms of spiritual support, and your expressions of love and support.

And all of you hospital people out there, lurking and never speaking up, you KNOW how grateful I am for your contributions! You're the ones who have delivered the goods, medically, much to our benefit. See you soon!

Dave & Ginny

p.s. On a more mundane front, I discovered something: If you can't bend your leg much (so you can't reach your foot), and you can't find your shoehorn, then a tablespoon makes a noble replacement. (Wash before returning to drawer.)

Friday, June 22, 2007 11:41 PM

I've had a mixed bag of things going on in my head and my life this week. It's odd, because we got that wonderful news last Monday, but I've not been jumping up and down for joy. It's just like "Okay, that's what's next. Dull thud."

So, what does THAT mean? Nothing. It's just odd.

Here are some of the week's events:

- We got the date for the next treatments: We start Monday July 2. Treatment that week, home the week of the 9th, treatment the week of the 16th, home the week of the 23rd.

- Had some solid accomplishments at work. (Today my manager said "You're back, aren't you.")

- Found that my leg incision has an infection; started treating it. Messy, annoying.

- Because the leg brace was pressing directly on the infection, I stopped wearing it. Risky; must be careful.

- Learned today (from my PT) how to go up & down stairs with crutches. This gives me a boatload of greater flexibility in getting around easily. Also pedaled vigorously on the PT's stationary bike to improve leg flexibility.

- Had some very, very stimulating meetings at work. It is indeed looking like a once-in-a-lifetime opportunity. How lucky is THAT?

- Researched and handled two insurance issues, to cope with the extremely tight money situation, which is about to get much tighter.

It feels, as they say in Boston, "bizaa" to have all these good things happening again at work, and then STOP it all (again) for a month to get more treatment. But I have to remind myself that I still have cancer and I choose to address it aggressively. Maybe that's why the week hasn't seemed thrilling – there's just a lot going on.

And after all, what are we committed to – good results, or having an exciting time along the way? Again, I remind myself that I have an aggressive cancer, which we're beating. It would be crazy to whine about not having enough excitement.

Ahoy, Davey-sitting brigade

Now that we know the schedule for IL-2, we know which weeks I'll be at home: the weeks of July 9 and July 23. Ginny is currently working Weds and Fridays, so if you're available for a half day or full day those dates, send me an email. I cannot say enough good things about the healing effect you folks had when you came and cared for me.

p.s. All you people on the "shrink the ulna met" team, good work: it's smaller AGAIN. We've canceled the radiation treatment it was going to get; may not need it soon.

Sunday, June 24, 2007 12:39 PM

For Round 2, a game worth playing

I got it! Yesterday Ginny and I were out enjoying the absolutely gorgeous day, truly happy to be alive in the day. I was thinking about my last post, about the sorta "dull thud" feeling that I have about Round 2, because "it's just more of the same." This time around, we already know I'm an Interleukin responder, so that mystery isn't there: I'm just gonna go get more of it. Compared to April's bold journey into the unknown, this is relatively ho-hum.

But I reminded myself that in our choice of language to describe our situation, we can have a substantial effect on how things turn out. In a way this is magical, but I've seen it often enough that I just accept it. I don't care whether I understand it. So, this time I've already created with my care team the goal of heading for "Club NED" – No Evidence of Disease; complete disappearance of all visible tumors. RIGHT NOW, this time around, by the end of Round 2 (early October).

But even with no evidence of disease, the medicos won't call it a cure because it can come back. (Truth in advertising, if you will.) That's largely because there are probably still little "met pellets" scattered all through the body, which can "wake up" or get activated, becoming new tumors years later. (My cancer is Grade 4, the most aggressive type. While learning about cancer months ago, I read that an aggressive tumor sends out zillions of invisible little "possible future met" particles, which lodge in various places throughout the body and may sit there for years. If something eventually triggers one of them to start growing, then presto, we now have a visible metastasis, aka "met.")

So yesterday, I got that I can create a great new super-goal: instead of just going for the predictable (no evidence of disease), let's go way beyond that: let's take on a goal that can't even be measured, and declare that we'll achieve THAT. And the goal is: We will transform my innards such that ALL of these pre-met pellets are GONE.

What a wild thing to do: We can take responsibility for achieving something (in reality), even though there's no way to tell! I assert that our medical services and providers have only begun to find out what Interleukin can achieve, in combination with a large number of people (you) focusing their energies on visualizing a radically healthy reality. And I assert that in this context, the nasty little pellets can simply unwrap whatever molecular bonds hold them together, and they can un-become what they are, and dissolve into the surrounding healthy tissue.

Obviously, this is not just about my case; what we create here will create a new future for every cancer patient today and into the future. So whaddaya think, people?? Are you in?

Monday, June 25, 2007 9:45 PM

We visited the orthopedist today for an evaluation of the June 7 leg surgery. The bone is mending great, she says.

Then her assistant exercised his sadistic streak by removing the staples from my incisions. Actually, the vast majority of it was no big deal – but the last couple were quite something. "I always save the worst ones for last," he says. Good thing for him!

Then they went to work on the infection that had started in the incision. THAT wasn't fun – but they say it's in much better shape now, and will be fine. (In the middle of that, through gritted teeth, I said to Ginny "After this is done I get ICE CREAM!" And I did – a banana cream pie Blizzard from Dairy Queen.)

Our next visit isn't until August 6, which is two full months after the surgery, and a week after our 7/28 concert. Sure hope it'll be fixed by THEN!

This weekend we saw the perfect bumper sticker for the recent messages here, about creating a game worth playing:

YOU ARE YOUR OWN FORTUNE COOKIE.

Amen.

Tuesday, June 26, 2007 12:10 PM

Boy, was THAT fun!

I sent around a note of celebration at work, and, disregarding all thought of embarrassment, told them about our raspberry party to celebrate my "drop dead date," and invited them to meet me and join in.

And what a site: at about 11:58, across our sea of cubicles, I saw heads coming from all directions.

When we did the raspberry it made quite a sound, and woke up the people who'd lost track of the time ... more heads popped up and came over, so we did it again.

Thank you so much for joining in this celebration! It marks the start of the work that remains, yet to be done. Let's go!

"This has been so important.
I've learned the true power of love and support.
I've learned that to go through something this hard alone
is not noble.

"We have to give of ourselves completely
to be open enough to receive all that comes back to us.
As your tumors shrink, we grow."

CaringBridge guestbook note
Teresa Palese, 6/19/07

Chapter 12: Understanding the Statistics We're Told

The statistics we read are often misleading. This can harm your outlook.

I'm not saying you should ignore evidence. To the contrary, when you're sizing up your options, you need the best possible information, and medical reports can be misleading.

Medically I was in trouble – I had tumors that were growing rapidly, tumors that often kill people. (You don't have to read ACOR long to know that's real.) But the statistics I found gave me an incomplete picture. Points to remember:

- Statistics are used as a "best guess" when we don't have certainty. The more you know about your case, the less applicable most statistics are.

- *The median isn't the message.* That's the title of an important article by eminent scientist and Pulitzer Prize winner Stephen Jay Gould. Diagnosed at age 41 with a nasty cancer, he learned that the median survival was eight months. He died 20 years later of something else. His article explains, with clear writing and scientific rigor, why the median's misleading.

- In fact, any single number is useless for understanding your odds. My friend Peter Schmidt is Vice President, Programs and Chief Information Officer, National Parkinson Foundation. Formerly an investment banker, he knows how to see through bad math. He says, "My advice for anyone who is told a single statistic about a disease is to recognize that you've been told nothing."

In my case, the best information available was "median survival 24 weeks," which means "half the people like you that we studied were dead in 24 weeks." That might be true (depending on what "people like you" means), but it still doesn't answer "What about the other half??"

In many cases the median isn't statistically appropriate, but researchers report it because it's the only number they have! You'd think the science journals would be sharper, but the fact that a number's been published is no guarantee of validity. Before taking a number seriously, dig into where it came from.

The Median is a Devil

The median is the most often, most severely misused and misunderstood statistic.

If you line up a set of numbers in order, the median is the middle one. It might be the same as others around it, or not – it's just the middle one. Think back to grade school, when the class lined up in alphabetical order: the middle kid's name might start with J or R or who knows.

In science, let's say you start a clinical trial with 11 patients, to see how long they live:

1	2	3	4	5	6	7	8	9	10	11

The middle one is #6, so when the sixth one dies, you can report the median for your study. And often, that's when scientists publish – without knowing how long the others live.

For instance, these three sets of 11 scores have the same median. In each set the middle score (the 6th value) is 2.

#	1	2	3	4	5	6	7	8	9	10	11
A:	1	1	1	1	1	2	5	10	30	60	80
B:	2	2	2	2	2	2	2	2	2	3	4
C:	0	0	0.1	0.2	0.3	2	2	3	5	8	9

See? *When you read the median, you have no idea about the other numbers.*

This is more than just a statistical gripe – it affects our ability to evaluate our options. When I saw "median survival 5.5 months" I got no information about whether anyone had lived longer. For that, you need another statistic – the range:

A: Median 2, range 1-80 (a huge range – but you can't tell that from the median)

B: Median 2, range 2-4 (note that 11 of the 13 people had exactly the same outcome, but you can't tell that from the median)

C: Median 2, range 0-9 (half the numbers are tiny – 6x smaller than the median – but you can't tell that from the median)

Discussing this in my ACOR cancer community I wrote, "That's a big deal! Does nobody publish papers characterizing the BEST outcomes? Why not show the whole curve?" Group leader Robin Martinez responded "good study reports DO include the range and will put in something like 'median 5.5 months (range 1-44+ months)' to indicate the top end has not yet been reached."

One more thing: before you even think about applying a study to your situation, you need to know how closely those people matched you. I know a guy who was told (before he was even drinking age) that he had six months to live. A wise fellow patient took him to a medical library and pointed out that those studies all included people who were retirement age. That was in the 1980s.

e-Patient take-aways:

- The median isn't the message. What's the complete set of numbers? Who was studied?

- Be informed by statistics, but don't be limited by them.

All the above came to light – because of my smart patient community – in my first weeks after diagnosis. So, from the beginning, I was liberated from worrying about the median: the reality for me was that no good data existed to predict my outcome.

Later, as I studied e-patient principles, I realized increasingly the importance of questioning the data we read. As you'll see in the following blog posts, and in the appendix, not everything we're told in the press is relevant or reliable – not even things we hear at medical conferences. Think critically; ask questions.

◆   ◆   ◆

In one of my first blog posts, I recognized that ordinary citizens can contribute important thoughts.

Saturday, October 27, 2007

Boston Kidney Cancer Association Conference

Yesterday I attended the Kidney Cancer Association's Boston "patient day." I wore my "Hey cancer! You picked the wrong guy" shirt. *(See Chapter 15.)* We got presentations from top Boston doctors in the field. My surgeon showed (with video [yech]) what's involved in kidney surgery, my oncologist talked about HDIL-2, and I learned a few new things about other treatments. Since kidney cancer often returns, it was a useful opportunity to learn about treatments I might want in the future. (My plan is to have a "lasting complete response," but I'm still interested in knowing stuff.)

Now, about my participation in the day. Now that I have this new lease on life, I'm doing and saying things that I might have inhibited in the past. (Yes, me.) The first speaker presented the same familiar statistics I've complained about in the past. Since they were nice enough to put a microphone right next to my chair, I hopped up to confirm with a truly authoritative source something I've long wanted confirmed. First I thanked the doctor, who's head of the BID program, and told people how bad off I'd been at first and how well I am now, so nobody would have the experience that I was just attacking this guy. I am GRATEFUL for his team's skill and knowledge. I asked a couple of detail questions, and then:

> Me: "My last question is about something that really affects families and patients who've just gotten a new diagnosis. The table you showed of median survival times – that's from the database of cases from 1976-1995, right?"

> Him: "That's correct."

Me: "And if I understand correctly, NONE of today's treatments were available at that time, right?"

Him: "That's correct."

Me: "So those figures have nothing to do with outcomes for someone who's diagnosed today, right?"

Him: "That's correct."

Me: "Well I WISH you guys would SAY that!"

I said it in a way that got some laughter – my point was that people who see those stats get a sense of the future that's simply wrong, and we don't need to do that. The thing is, that table shows up everywhere – it was featured in an oncology nurse training program experienced by classmate/guestbooker Peggy Weber just 17 months ago. And nobody ever says "This is NOT what you can expect today – a lot has changed since then"!

This was underscored during a Q&A session in the afternoon, when someone raised his hand and started by saying "I was diagnosed 13 years ago…" Later, I raised my hand, and said: "I'm glad he said that, because to listen to the statistics this morning, you'd think that wasn't possible. What people need to understand – especially people who are new to the diagnosis – is that statistics apply to POPULATIONS, and they don't tell you a thing about YOUR outcome."

"There's a limit," I said, "to how useful statistics are for understanding your situation." I paused and made a fateful choice to continue: "I'm going to get a little bit crude here, to make the point in a way you won't forget: The average person has one ball and one tit! … It's true, but it tells you nothing about YOU."

Well, there were reactions. A British guy at my table almost fell off his chair laughing, there was tentative laughter around the room (mostly from women), and the session leader (a social worker) said, "I've forgotten what my next point was going to be."

142

Monday, October 29, 2007

About those statistics

Thanks to all those who sent me private notes about my anatomy/ statistics remarks. :)

I want to answer an aspect of the note my mom wrote. I'm clear that the people who present these stats are doing so because that's the way it's done in the medical profession: reliably done studies are the most respected, and thus the most respectable to present. Neither that doctor, nor the professionals who put together the flyer that nurse Peggy Weber received, were being reckless by citing those stats, at least not intentionally, and not as far as current professional standards require.

And that's where I want to change things. Friday was specifically intended to be a patient-facing conference, a "Patient Day," but its content was often (not always) very technical, and few of the topics were from the patient's point of view, except patients who've become very advanced in their medical knowledge.

What these skilled caregivers need to realize, in addition to all they know, is that WE need information and coaching that fits OUR situation – which is different from taking what interests clinicians and simplifying it to the patient's level. And that starts by asking patients (ordinary ones) what's on their mind.

It's similar to something that came up at a Beth Israel Deaconess hospital board dinner I attended two weeks ago. When they asked for areas of improvement, I mentioned the problem of silos (information that is available within one part of the organization, but not shared with other parts): "We all know about silos of knowledge, but I found there are also silos of treatment. In my first admission, I had two conditions to be watched at the same time: my kidney surgery and my leg (which had not yet broken). The people involved with the kidney didn't know beans about my leg situation, and vice versa; when I mentioned this to several people at the hospital, they all said it's not a problem.

"Well...," I said, "it IS a problem. SOMEbody's got to be responsible for the whole patient, or I'm left wondering what they might be overlooking and what I might need to know that I don't know." Medicine (at least at some care centers) is striding strongly toward the patient's perspective. It's the same shift that businesses in general have been doing: moving toward a customer orientation. But in both the "silos" issue and the information available at a "patient day," medicine as I'm experiencing it hasn't yet made the fundamental brain shift to see things from our point of view. They'll get there – and you and I can be voices for it. Speak up!

Chapter 13: Interleukin, Round 2

July 3 – September 12, 2007

Tuesday, July 3, 2007 7:38 AM

I started the second round of Interleukin yesterday, and so far, it's uneventful!

This time we got a room at the end of the hall. Much quieter. I slept like a proverbial baby.

I just finished getting the third dose of Interleukin. After the first dose I did a splendid rendition of Le Grand Barfe, but not after the late-night dose. I'm feeling well and very much enjoying the opportunity to sleep for long hours.

Ginny headed home overnight, to care for herself (and the, ahem, cats...). It's nice to feel that things are predictable enough to do that.

p.s. VERY glad the Red Sox decided to start looking like a real baseball team, last night!

Tuesday, July 3, 2007 7:42 PM

Well, friends and family, it's Ginny here.

Dave is feeling lousy this evening. He has had 4 treatments so far and the GI symptoms are back along with the chills. We were told a frequent symptom that occurs with the 2nd round is aching joints. A bit of that is starting as well. But what I'm focusing on is the "death toll" of those little mets. We are planning to take a wheelchair ride to the other end of the building to see fireworks tomorrow night. HAPPY FOURTH of JULY everyone.

Ginny (and Dave)

Wednesday, July 4, 2007 8:56 AM

I'm not having joint pain – it's overall aches and pains. I wanted it to go away on its own, but it didn't, so around 9pm I gave up the tough guy routine and asked for meds.

Meanwhile, this week, as treatment continues, my blood pressure is dropping again, as it did during the second April week. At this stage they want it to be >85 (e.g. 85/62), and my last few readings have trended down from 131 to 86. So I have a concern that it'll be below 85 next time and the next dose will be held back.

Wednesday, July 4, 2007 4:11 PM

I just finished receiving dose #7 (yay!). Midday they gave me additional fluid, and the BP popped back up to 92.

Friday, July 6, 2007 7:37 PM

Hi all, Ginny here. I left Dave yesterday a.m. in a very groggy state. He has been rather incoherent on the phone since then. This is one of the side effects of the IL-2 that we heard about but hadn't experienced before. His daughter Lindsey visited last night and this evening and said he mostly slept while she was there and was still confused about many things. The confusion starts clearing up soon after the IL-2 stops, from what I remember being told by the docs.

Dave told me that he had 10 doses and they were stopping at that number. He should get home tomorrow or Sunday. I suspect Sunday will be the day.

Sunday, July 8, 2007 10:24 PM

We've been very, very resting today. Got home before 1 (pm), let myself relax, fell asleep, ate something yummy around suppertime, and rested this evening. It was LOUSY trying to get rest/be rested in the hospital.

Folks, I declare that I intend to use this week for recovery: to rest and be in balance by the time I return Monday 7/16 for my final week.

146

Tuesday, July 10, 2007 10:15 PM

Sleep, glorious sleep... sleep, sleep, take another nap. I had no idea how much sleep I needed! A mere 36 hrs of it and I'm feeling much better. (Soooooooo many dreams in there, too. So much of life's secrets to explore in pillow land.)

Side effect update

Nausea etc.: it's here, at about 1/3 of April's level. Unsettling but tolerable. Keeps me uneasy; I'm never far from my "buckets."

Skin flakes are here early! So many that I've got to keep (carefully) picking them away from my eyes! As in late April, I discovered them today in full bloom on my face by looking in the mirror. You never know.

Sunday, July 15, 2007 1:49 PM

It's been a roller coaster weekend. Saturday morning was stinkin' rotten, based on how I felt. This morning was great, then not. Suede intervened with brilliant advice via email, which represenced the Roxanna Ward song she sings, "Remember who you are." I cried and let some things go, cried more, let more things go. I feel complete, somewhat ouchy but free to love.

This week had been so good – generally on the upward trend. My Tuesday knee hurt hasn't improved but it hasn't been a constant pain. I've returned to wearing the brace, which I'd discontinued with the doctor's ok because it was squeezing my infected incision. (The infection's much better.) The week's weather's been great. At home I've been able to get to the bottom of the billing/budgeting pile, so on Thursday afternoon Ginny and I realized we could take a run down to Cape Cod, which turned into an impromptu visit with sister Suede, who also had a time slot open up unexpectedly.

Then: AAUUUGGGHHHHH – WHERE'S MY HAIR??? Having had no hair loss side effect, suddenly I seem to have 1/3 as much as I used to! And MAN does it look ooooogly/scraggly! I realized that

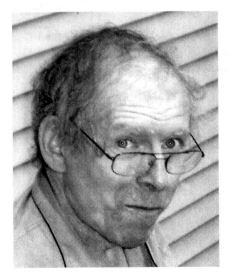

I'd started avoiding mirrors, and when I suddenly caught a full view, it was A A U U G G G H H H H H! I have a see-thru coat of light head fur. NOT IN MY PLAN! I know many of you have experienced this, more than I. It's just that I thought I ALREADY KNEW EVERYTHING I'D HAVE TO FACE! I thought I'd gotten to the top of the mountain and could see everything there was to see.

But no. This week, all the side effects have been different from before. And who knows what it'll be next week. (The untransformed way of saying that is "It never stops, does it?? Just one damn thing after another," all with a strong tone of injustice.) Overnight Suede brought all this together brilliantly, as she's done before. It bears repeating: "...allow yourself that honestly, when that is what is present – like Buddha says, acceptance of what is now. Have the feeling, watch it, notice it, name it, then let it go. Over and over again. Once the attachment leaves, the struggle disappears. I am also a firm believer that acknowledging those feelings when they surface and letting them 'be' and then releasing them creates space to be in transformation ..."

So, yeah, I am TIRED of having an unpredictable life, I am TIRED of the taste of the hospital food (which ain't that bad), I am TIRED of not walking, I am TIRED of not knowing what's going to happen, TIRED of so many things. And, any attachment to those feelings won't serve me in any away. They are my human experience, and they bring me no power: they don't leave me freed up to do whatever needs doing. It's miraculous that I can acknowledge them and let go and become free to be effective – starting with Monday morning's 8 a.m. appointment with the orthopedist. And then – the final week of IL-2! I love you all – thank you for being here.

— Dave

Monday, July 16, 2007 11:30 AM

Hi, Ginny here. We arrived bright and early for our appointment with Dr. Anderson, orthopedist, to check on Dave's slowly healing incision. Dave had a lot of anxiety overnight and had a hard time sleeping, so he is zonked out here at the hospital. I read him all the CaringBridge guest entries and I was the one in tears. Thanks gang for making me cry (I think). I am sure Dave will give you more news as the day and week continue.

Thursday, July 19, 2007 10:53 AM

Hi everyone – Here it is Thursday morning and suddenly things are buzzing right along! For the first time this week, I got a solid 5-hour stretch of sleep, and my goodness what a difference THAT makes. Until then, all I had was patches of 10-15 minutes at a time. I have been a tired cowpoke, taking YOUR advice to just let myself rest, thank you.

I've learned that this week is indeed the END of my IL-2 treatments. (Only in rare cases does someone get more than this.) I'll repeat the waiting period before the final CAT scans, and then after that, we kick back and just have scans every few months for long-term follow-up.

In other words, boys & girls, we are pretty much at the (successful) completion of my entire treatment for RCC (renal cell carcinoma). Meanwhile, Dr. Anderson says I may be walking unassisted in a few weeks.

Saturday, July 21, 2007 11:36 PM

I AM GONNA BE SO FREAKIN' GLAD TO BE OUT OF HERE!

The planned exit date is no surprise (Sunday, July 22, my Mom's birthday!). But what is a surprise is the realization that this is basically the end of the planned HDIL treatment plan. I am like DONE – there's no standard planned "return for more in x months."

So this is it, folks. I am LEAVING HERE! We'll have scans some months down the road, for years 'n' years, even AFTER they say "N.E.D.!"

Thursday, July 26, 2007 9:14 PM

The past couple of days have been another(!) snowflake fest. For the second time this week my face is sloughing (what a gross thing to say) and my hair is doing the Great Scott thing again.

Meanwhile my legs and feet have developed what I call alligator skin. The "tiles" aren't as apparent as on a real gator, but the skin is that dry and in need of lotion.

But my digestion this week has been well behaved: no emergencies at all. I'm very happy about that, and I'm almost happy to trade it for the snowfall.

Interwoven with the medical drama was the financial drama of owning an unsold house back in Minnesota, with $3,000/month of carrying costs, while the housing market hit the skids. When we finally got an offer it was for much less than we owed on the mortgage. Incredibly, my superstar singer sister Suede booked herself into a local music hall and held a July 28 benefit concert with fund drive. Here's my post from the next day. (You should buy her CDs.)

Sunday, July 29, 2007 2:58 PM

Oh my goodness, oh my goodness, oh my goodness. What a NIGHT!

It was unbelievably touching and moving to see so many of you. And I honestly think it was the best Suede show I've ever seen.... and that's going some.

The financial proceeds were beyond my expectations, though the grin on Suede's face today suggests that she's entirely accustomed to producing unbelievable results.

I was equally touched by the fact that my mom and sister Amy came up from Maryland. It was just SO GOOD to have them here, and to be so well supported. And my primary physician, Danny Sands, was there with his wife. They had to leave at intermission – but they didn't: 'We came for Dave, but we stayed for Suede.' It seems they were blown away by the first act, and couldn't decide which CDs to buy, so they stayed to hear more songs after the intermission.

We're humbled and blessed to have received so much support. We're thinking seriously about what to do that's now possible and wasn't possible a week ago. Certainly we're going to make some choices to reduce the risk in our near-term financial future, and some choices to support well-being. Considering what our world looked like a week ago, this is all darn-near miraculous.

And triple-thanks to ringleader Suede, creator of miracles. What a show! Thank you, all.

Friday, August 3, 2007 10:34 PM

Holy cow, you guys – I am humbled (happily) by your comments this week, and in a way I'm reminded who I am and who we all are: remarkable creators of the world we live in.

I've had a few days of feeling isolated for some reason, isolated and powerless, complaining about my body (particularly my leg) not cooperating with my wishes. How's that for idiotic? :-) That's the human system for ya: turn your back on it for a moment and it's up to its old tricks again.

Yet at the same time, although I don't remember it as an overall plan, what I was doing this week was much clearer evidence that the drive to create was intact, and not at all consistent with the mopey state my head was in:

1. Two visits to the physical therapist. (My leg continues to be

my major hold-back...grrr! All the muscles have atrophied for 5-6 months. I am so tired of crutches and impaired mobility.)

2. Began pro-actively creating what use we'll make of the proceeds of the benefit concert Suede held for us a week ago.

3. Resumed participation in my chorus as a full member.

4. As part of #1 and #2, boldly inquired at the local fitness club, and discovered their prices are much less than I'd expected... and, gulping hard, signed up for (leg) strength training with a personal trainer. (VERY hard to do that, but I used what I've learned from you about accepting nurturance.)

5. Kept open the option of staying home another week, if that's what seems right.

6. Did a half day of work today, at the office, testing the waters.

What all this says to me is, my mood is a rotten indicator of reality .:-) And it shows the power of not honoring my mood, but instead creating from nothing.

Dave

Monday, August 6, 2007 9:28 PM

Dem bones

First, we visited Dr. Anderson the bone doc to find out the status of this blasted leg. Answer: the femur has healed well! I (finally!) don't have to see her again for three months!

I finally have a clear picture that my mission, at last, is just to get the leg muscles strong enough to resume their usual job.

I see the PT again Tuesday and the trainer Wednesday. She wrote instructions for them on getting my muscles strengthened without overdoing it, busting a tendon, etc.

Hey Meester – want to see peectures of my body?

My innards, specifically – bones and guts. Today I exercised my right to get a copy of all the images they've ever taken of me – femur x-rays, CT scans, everything. It fills 6 CDs.

BUT, it comes with image viewing software that has no similarity to ordinary photo viewing software. It'll take a bit of work in their Help file to understand how to use it.

Part of me is eager to find the juicy original images that showed the first tumor evidence, and then gloat about how the lesions aren't there anymore. But another part of me hopes the imaging will be so obscure that there's nothing really for an untrained eye to see.

(Repeat after me.... "It is what it is, whether I know it or not.... it is what it is, whether I know it or not...")

Energy level

I phoned the oncologist's office today and said, "I've been having a triad of symptoms: more tired than I'd expect, losing weight (10# since last hospitalization), and appetite not back to normal."

They called this afternoon and asked if I can come in tomorrow (Tuesday), their clinic day. I said sure. (Some of my symptoms are consistent with a thyroid problem that's common after HDIL-2 treatment..... grrr, says me – why didn't y'all tell me to watch out for it?? I've been staying out of work because of this energy level issue!)

Tuesday, August 7, 2007 8:02 PM

Bottom line of today's visit is that the blood tests all came back negative: no thyroid problem, no anemia.

So, at this point, the leading explanation for all my yawns and 10# weight loss is simply (duh) that I just had an IL-2 treatment. Both complaints are well within the (wide) range of common reactions to IL-2, the folks said today.

And "what's next" remains unchanged: get the scheduled CAT

scans next Monday, have the team review them, and meet to get the results on Monday 8/20.

I DON'T LIKE WAITING! No surprise there; breathe, see it, let it go, breathe.

I'll just continue feeding myself and giving my body all the rest it wants.

Dave

Friday, August 10, 2007 9:26 PM

House news (dare we think it?)

Remember the couple from Idaho who made an offer on our Minnesota house? It was contingent on selling their house, and we weren't surprised when the months went by with no further news. Well, suddenly, although the contract had expired, the realtor HAS a buyer now, ready to close Sept. 15.

Progress and progression

Monday, the bone doc wrote to the PT that he's to move me along from 2 crutches to 1 crutch to cane. (She won't see me again for months.) The next day, based on his observations, the PT authorized me to use 1 crutch when away from home, and if I want, use no crutches at home as long as I'm walking between things that I can reach out to if needed (a chair back, a tabletop, etc.). But this time around I have *no* interest in moving faster than my leg is ready for, so I'm being more conservative than those instructions. I must say, I'm moving around better than ever (Ginny says so) and I wanna keep it that way. And when that thigh muscle gets tired out, I put it on ice – it works.

Work

I know some of you are going to strenuously object to this item. Just hear me when I say I've heard your concerns and I'm paying attention, not ignoring you.

A week ago I was a snooze monster, going from nap to nap with sometimes just an hour between them. That's over. Yesterday I was actually getting restless, looking for something to do. I got word of a problem at the office so I went in for a while. As I worked on it, I realized "I'm back." The same applied when I went in today. Also, my weight is climbing slowly, which I take as a good sign: both the fatigue and the weight loss are gone.

Sooo.....this week is spontaneously full of all good news, so far. Some is tentative, but I know what to do with that: latch on and create a result!

Wednesday, August 15, 2007 10:57 PM

The physical therapist says I can now walk with just a cane, when I need one, instead of crutches.

I had a good day at work, a good evening with chorus, a nice haircut and some very good news:

1. I got tired of my cancer-hair being unsolveably weird, so I went and got a buzz cut. Specifically with "#0A Red" clippers. I'm not totally skinheaded, but believe me you can now tell the shape of my skull.

2. THE DEAL ON OUR HOUSE CAME THROUGH. We're closing Sept. 6 – just 3 weeks from now! We will once again own just one house!

As I've said before, the sale price is a lot lower than what we owe on the mortgage, so we'll have to bring a lot of cash to the closing, just to get out from under. And you know what is making that work? At least 2/3 of the necessary amount was raised by the extraordinary benefit that Suede put together and so many of you supported.

I don't know what it takes to qualify as a miracle, but it's pretty darn close when, within a few weeks, the benefit happens and then we get a call that the expired offer has been renewed, and it all comes together.

What the hell, everyone: MIRACLES! Why not spend our whole lives creating 'em?

THANK YOU – NO KIDDING.

G'night.

Sunday, August 19, 2007 8:01 PM

Milestones on the road to recovery

Yesterday I went back to the very beginning of the Journal and started re-reading. Considering what the world looked like in January, this is a wonderful place to be, eh?

1. Department of Transportation

I'm now walking only with the cane (or unassisted), so this weekend we did the following amazing things:

1. Returned the scooter to the rental place (woohoo!)
2. Boxed up the Hugo Rolling Walker to put it into storage
3. Put the crutches back in the coat closet

2. Department of Partnership

This morning as I walked past Ginny in the living room, SHE asked ME to get her something from the kitchen. It's the first time since January the request has gone in that direction (instead of me asking her). Also, within my limits, I assisted her with several tasks during the day.

Tomorrow morning there's a 7am fitness appointment, starting the work week. At 2pm we have the post-CAT-scan meeting with the oncology team.

Monday, August 20, 2007 5:46 PM

"Extraordinary" results

That's what Dr. McDermott and super-nurse Kendra Bradley said today, presenting the findings from last week's scans: "Extraordinary." "NOT typical." And more good things that I was too excited to remember. (Believe me, when you're in a situation like this, there's a LOT on the line as you wait for the words to come out of the team's mouths.)

This time they were willing to share some quantitative information with us. Apparently they use some measure of the total surface area of all the lesions they're following. In March, the number was 38.18. Now it's 6.25. In other words, the tumors are 83% gone. The largest remaining one is 0.9″ x 0.5″. MAN is this good to hear. And we've still got another month to go, for the immunotherapy to bear more results. That's no small issue (in my mind), because in the first round, the lesions shrank 50% between the first and second CAT scans. N.E.D.! NO METS! TOTALLY CLEAN AND VITAL BEING! Yes.

p.s. Kendra said "Remember, early on? I said you're going to make me a star." How's THAT for a powerful expectation from a key team member??

Sunday, August 26, 2007 1:37 PM

The cost of treatment

Ever wondered how much this is all costing? Frankly, during these months I've preferred not to think about it. But now I'm willing to look. I received a 10-page bill from Beth Israel Deaconess for my July 2 week of Interleukin. I was astounded to see the cost of that single week. The amount I owe is just $500; my insurance company, Harvard Pilgrim Health Care, paid $87,948.12. For one week.

The main cost is the Interleukin itself. Hold onto your hats: $7,032 per dose. I had 11 doses that week, which accounts for $77,352 of the total. Room & board, semi-private, $712/night x 6 = $4300, brings it to $81,652. The rest is mostly lab tests, because most of the meds are pretty cheap: Naproxen (Aleve) 36c; ranitidine (Zantac) 36c; acetaminophen 18c.

One thing that inspires me about Beth Israel Deaconess is that they're one of the hospitals that still provides care (the same quality of care) to everyone regardless of ability to pay. I don't know how they manage that, but it's inspiring.

Tuesday, August 28, 2007 6:24 PM

More milestones today:

- It's the first day that I didn't use a handicapped spot at work (or anywhere else). I parked in the regular parking lot and walked in & out of the building, like ordinary folk.

- Haven't used my cane in 2 days. (Mind you, I carry it with me (folded up), but I haven't used it.)

- Physical therapist says we'll be finished in 2 weeks.

- In a few minutes my guys are showing up for our first quartet rehearsal in forever.

Dave

Wednesday, September 12, 2007 7:02 PM

Quickie before going to chorus –

I was talking to supernurse Kendra today, about future care (beyond the clinical trial), and she asked if I wanted to know the results of this week's scan. "Well," I sez to myself, "it sounds like they don't figure I'll need to see a counselor after getting the news." So I said sure.

They have the target lesions – 4 mets in my left lung. Those are the ones they've been watching and measuring. Those are stable since a month ago – no change. I told her I wanted them GONE, but she said (I'll paraphrase) to shut up, because stable is very good with RCC.

"It's all about the trend, the direction things are going," she said. "This is good."

Then she said "How about this?" and read me something else from the radiologist's report: "NON-target lesion in lower RIGHT lobe is massively reduced."

Then she said "I don't think I've ever seen 'massively' in a report. That's an interesting word." (Remember, this is a profession where the top doc got so excited that he said I'm "not typical." So "massively" is pretty cool.)

So I'm feeling very cool and powerful tonight. And it means Monday's meeting really will be about creating the future ("What can we do now"), because we've already got the basic status news.

Now I go sing. Yay.

Chapter 14: When I Leave the World Behind

Sunday, April 11, 2010

As I worked on this book the fear, the pain, of facing death came back vividly. It was unexpected – I guess that's because when I escaped and got free, I pretty much put all that in the attic. But today it came back. And I'm glad, because I want this book to connect with people in situations like mine: facing death.

As I worked on the Hope section, I read Jerome Groopman MD's book *The Anatomy of Hope*. It's filled with stories of being with patients as they faced probable death, and the physician's journey of learning to help them deal with it.

I cried as I recalled facing my own death. It was accentuated by recent events:

- Fellow kidney cancer patient Rick Schleider died last month.

- My classmate Don Levinstone lost his fight with pervasive lung cancer last month.

- Last week my dear singer-sister Suede's longtime companion dog Angel died. Angel was a miracle dog, an abused stray who lived on a highway median for months before being rescued. Suede adopted her and gave her a life she never would have known. The loss is hard on her.

- Today's CBS Sunday Morning had a segment on children who lose a parent. (5% do, before age 15.) The family photos and the footage of the children's words, their loss, brought me back to the thought of leaving my family behind.

And that brought me back to my own father's death in 2005, when I lived a thousand miles away. Traveling to see him wasn't easy. The last time I left him in the care facility I said I'd be back soon and kissed his forehead. His last words to me were "That will be nice." All signs were that the end was near, and it was.

That night I attended the annual concert of my sister Amy's excellent Sweet Adelines chorus, The Pride of Baltimore. The headline act was Wheelhouse, a champion quartet whose signature song is "When I Leave the World Behind." Irving Berlin's beautiful lyrics flooded me; I sat there with tears running down my face, thinking of my dad's departure from this world.

Today that song came back to me as I heard the children talk. I found Wheelhouse's performance on YouTube, and found myself sobbing with feelings I hadn't touched in three years, a much needed catharsis. (If you search for "Wheelhouse" and "When I Leave the World Behind" on YouTube, you'll find it. The handheld video is shaky at first but it settles down.) The song's lyrics are on the next page.

I'm so glad to still be alive, alive to keep loving those things for a few more years. Thanks to all of you who were with me then, and thanks to all of you who work today to make a world of better healthcare.

Laugh, Sing, and Eat Like a Pig

When I Leave the World Behind

Irving Berlin, 1915

I know a millionaire
Who's burdened down with care
A load is on his mind
He's thinking of the day
When he must pass away
And leave his wealth behind
I haven't any gold
To leave when I grow old
Somehow it passed me by
I'm very poor but still
I'll leave a precious will
When I must say good-bye

[Refrain:]
I'll leave the sunshine to the flowers
I'll leave the springtime to the trees
And to the old folks, I'll leave the mem'ries
Of a baby upon their knees
I'll leave the night time to the dreamers
I'll leave the songbirds to the blind
I'll leave the moon above
To those in love
When I leave the world behind

To every wrinkled face
I'll leave a fireplace
To paint their fav'rite scene
Within the golden rays
Scenes of their childhood days
When they were sweet sixteen
I'll leave them each a song
To sing the whole day long
As toward the end they plod
To ev'ry broken heart
With sorrow torn apart
I'll leave the love of God

[Refrain:]
I'll leave the sunshine to the flowers
I'll leave the springtime to the trees
And to the old folks, I'll leave the mem'ries
Of a baby upon their knees
I'll leave the night time to the dreamers
I'll leave the songbirds to the blind
I'll leave the moon above
To those in love
When I leave the world behind

Chapter 15: Recovery

September 14, 2007 – January 30, 2008

Sunday, September 16, 2007 3:09 PM

A thank-you note (The ultimate "department of transportation" update)

I just had the experience of receiving a truly special gift from all of you. I went for a mile-long walk on this beautiful almost-fall day! And I experienced it as a direct gift from those who supported me in staying alive. I've always enjoyed the approach of fall, but never as much as I'm enjoying this one. So we took Ginny's granddaughter Lilly for a walk in the almost-woods at the bottom of our hill. (There's wetland and woods there, with a paved path about 10 feet off the road.)

We walked a mile. And it was SUCH a pleasure to be able to do so. And I had the long-forgotten experience of identifying what type of wildflower or tree we were walking past ... I re-experienced what it was like to be a Boy Scout. I hope you really get what a wonderful thing it is that you've given us.

The Oncology visit (Monday)

As promised, I wore the "Hey cancer!" shirt.

We positioned ourselves in the "meet the doctors" room such that I was behind the curtain and Ginny wasn't. So as each of them walked in, they greeted Ginny and then turned to greet me and got, well, a surprise.

Even Mister Top Dog Doctor had a broad grin on his face.

I asked for medication to treat my severe depression. (It's a JOKE, people. Work with me here.) They declined.

They said: until further notice I'll get scans every 12 weeks. For now, there's nothing more to do.

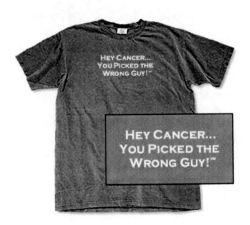

Supernurse Kendra gave me a printout of the full radiology report, so I could see where it says "massively reduced." It also mentioned a lytic lesion (lytic = bony; this is the one inside the skull). I said "I thought that was gone!" and they said that once the bone gets reshaped by a met, it stays that shape, even after the tumor goes bye-bye.

We said goodbye until the October Kidney Cancer Association conference in Cambridge, where they're presenting and I'm attending.

We stopped in at the cancer gift shop to show the manager my shirt. She went nuts over it and I suspect by now she's already called the maker up here in Cow Hampshire. (Not many cows left, actually – they've all been replaced by migrants from Massachusetts.)

Scan data

Tonight I went online and went back through all my scan and x-ray results (don't I love PatientSite!). Data geek that I may be, I had never put it all together. What emerges is quite a picture of the mets that they tracked. I got something of a chill when I put the whole picture together, and saw what was going on before we intervened.

You may recall that this clinical trial tracked four specific "target lesions" (mets). On the first scan on January 5, lesion #2 was the largest, at 30 mm x something.

When they did the pre-study scan in March, that one had grown to 41x33 mm. But it was no longer largest – lesion #1 had surged into first place, at 43x39. In other words, the nasties was growin' pretty rapidly.

Am I grateful again for the shoulder pain and x-ray that led to the early discovery? You betcha. The aggressive growth is consistent with my disease being Grade 4, the most aggressive grade. And the presence of a 33x25 met inside a muscle is rare except in the most aggressive cancers, they said.

Here's how met #1 progressed:

- 43x39 on Mar 21

- 37x35 in the May scan (after first round of IL-2 in April)

- 29x23 in the June scan

- 22x13 in the August scan (after the second round of IL-2 in July)

- 12x13 in the Sept. scan.

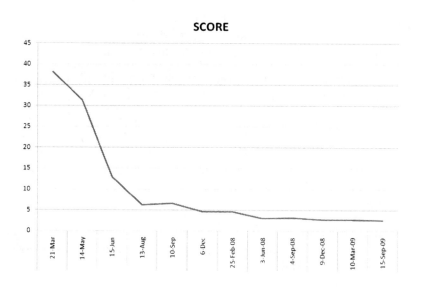

SCORE

In their "scoring system," that met went from 16.77 points down to 1.56. Woohoo!

Total score at each scan:

- 38.18 in March (pre-IL-2)
- 31.29 in May
- 12.89 in June (!!)
- 6.25 in August
- 6.6 in Sept (negligible change, they say: I'm good).

Total reduction: 83%. Woo-BLEEPING-hoo! (And it ain't over; that's just the most recent data.)

Sunday, September 30, 2007 1:36 PM

FABULOUS early-fall day. GLORIOUS cool air. And baseball is in the air, as we New Englanders get ready for the playoffs.

Philosophy

1. A signature block that I used to use:

> "Don't ask yourself what the world needs. Ask yourself what makes you come alive, and go do that, because what the world needs is people who are alive." – Gil Bailie

AMEN! And we don't just mean "still breathing," we mean ALIVE, fulfilled, vital, self-expressed, full of joy. JOY!

2. Two years ago I wrote to a good friend's daughter (she calls me uncle): "What do you think about responsibilities and freedom and joy, hm? What gives you joy? What feels like freedom, to you? Do responsibilities seem like a great burden to you or just part of life or non-existent or what?"

Do YOU know where you're going? If not, you run the risk of a danger reported to us by the one and only Yogi Berra: "You've got to be very careful if you don't know where you're going, because you might not get there."

Sunday, October 21, 2007 8:38 PM

WE WON! Yesterday was barbershop chorus competition. We won! New England champions (plus eastern Canada) for the 9th year in a row. We've been working hard to improve the quality of our sound, and having seen the DVD, I'm very pleased with the performance we put on. This means that during July 4th week, I get to go to International in Nashville, the world championships of men's barbershop singing.

Friday, November 16, 2007 9:30 PM

A quick note to let you know that things are great. My gait is almost back to completely normal. (A month ago I could only stand for a minute or two without sitting.) My job is going great. My romance is at least as good as ever. My quartet has a chance of gaining an excellent new coach. On Monday my chorus lays down the first two tracks of the new CD that will be released next year.

I submitted my patient empowerment outline to the volunteer office at my hospital, and got an interested response. (No follow-up yet, but that'll come.)

This is turning out to be a Fall that was very much worth coming back for. I love my life.

Wednesday, November 21, 2007 11:36 PM

These are a few of my favorite things

One of my blessings is the wonderful Dr. Danny Sands, my PCP, who wrote me the other day with these splendid words of advice: "Since the previous orders that I gave you at the time of your diagnosis – to eat as much as you like – have expired and you haven't, it is time to reconsider."

Alas, no more heeding that diet card titled "How to increase your caloric intake." Oh darn. The next day he wrote and said "One more thing: have a wonderful Thanksgiving. You have many things for which to be thankful."

That sank in. That night on my drive home I was singing along with my chorus's Christmas training CD (the baritone part on one channel, the other parts on the other channel), and I was thinking about inviting my neighbors to our concert on 12/15. For an instant I thought of mentioning to them that this is the Christmas I didn't know if I'd see. And instantly I was in tears – the first time in months that this has really sunk in. I really might have been dead & gone by now.

It all seems so long ago ... but I realized that this all started only 10-1/2 months ago. My NEXT annual physical is finally coming up (that's why I had the email exchange with the doctor). My treatment ended in late July – just 6-1/2 months after the diagnosis, and nearly 4 months ago.

Singing

You'll recall that in February the good doctor told me NOT to give up singing to conserve energy. "You do not want to start dropping life activities that you love," he said.

Well, I kept singing, and now I love it more than ever. I've relaxed, my singing is freer and more open, I'm expressing myself facially more than ever (less inhibited), and that makes me a better performer. I've continued moving from the back corner of the risers – now I'm down to the second row, close to center, which is a wonderfully fun place to be. [My dream since I first sang has been to earn my way up to being a Front Row Guy (wooooooo!).]

Monday, December 10, 2007 2:58 PM

Greetings from wireless in the doctor's office! And so, in the game of beating cancer, our winning continues! The lung mets are now 12% of the baseline measures in March.

So we continue – next follow-up scan is in 3 months. We have more work to do, my people – if we produce another 30% drop in 3 months, it'll be down to 8.6%, and then the tumor might as well just give up and go away!

I told Ginny yesterday that my best Christmas present, on Christmas morning, will be that I get to wake up on Christmas morning.

Sunday, December 30, 2007 3:33 PM

As my year with cancer draws to a close

We're in Provincetown for Suede's annual Dec. 30 "New Year's Eva with the Diva" show. It's odd, returning to the place where the story started a year ago. Three days later I had that x-ray, and a day later got the call saying "There's something in your lung."

I was sick then, and I'm not sick now, even though there are still tumors in me. I have a different view of life now, but more than that, I have a radically different view of cancer. As part of declaring this year complete, I'm going to lay out that new view.

♦   ♦   ♦

On Feb 3, in one of the earliest journal posts, I said:

> Some of you know that I realized last week that success in this journey doesn't require a complete disappearance of the tumors. (Disappearance is my goal, of course, but I've learned that many people simply stop the disease in its tracks so it never gets worse, or shrinks and stays that way. That would be fine with me: I'd be happy to feel this way for the next 20-30 years!)

I then quoted an MD (a kidney cancer patient himself) from my www.acor.org kidney cancer email group, saying "...[increasingly] cancer is being looked at as a chronic disease, much like diabetes, asthma, congestive heart failure, etc." I haven't had a drop of treatment for 5 months now, but the prolonged immune response is continuing – the lesions are 30% smaller than September.

Yesterday I asked the ACOR mailing list how long it may take for a "complete response" to appear (disappearance of all visible tumors). In the response I got, there was another piece of unexpected news:

> Dave, ongoing and/or delayed responses do happen with

IL-2. No one really knows how to "credit" these responses since they can happen so long after medication stops. However, since most patients haven't had any other treatment in between, it seems clear that IL-2 can indeed have a delayed response for some reason. Keep hoping for that complete response (or a permanent partial response, which we have also seen – and which we suspect means tumors that are completely dead but still present in the body).

Oh really?? So even if I have visible tumors on my CT scans, they might be dead? I'm reminded again of something we observed many times this year: reality is what it is, regardless of what we think. All mental stress and suffering arises in our *reactions* to what's so. We have complete choice in how we are about our circumstances.

More than anything else, I'd like to see this realization spread far and wide, available to people and families who are just getting their first cancer news: **it's not necessarily a death sentence.** Learn everything you can, ask many questions, don't assume any one person knows everything. And, most of all, be the master of your own life, however long it may last.

I'm not saying there's no such thing as being sick from cancer or dying from cancer. Back in May, an ACOR post said this:

Do you realize how lucky we are to have ANY cure rate at all for RCC? Stage IV lung cancer, breast cancer, and colon cancer are routinely terminal. Treatment can only delay death for those cancers; their patients are often in ongoing treatment that vastly reduces quality of life.

My point is that however long you last, you can be the master of your own life. We humans have the power to shift the world's conversation about anything – even cancer, even death.

Thursday, January 24, 2008 7:34 PM

My leg x-ray last week shows that my femur is finally growing replacement bone.

Recently my boss suggested we walk up the 3 flights of stairs from lunch. I've done it before, but this time my hands were full so no railing. I was winded at the top, but I did it.

This past week I regained the ability to put my pants on while standing on one leg at a time, without leaning against anything. A real milestone.

Wednesday, January 30, 2008 11:21 PM

Declaring the year complete

One year ago tonight, 1/30/07, I posted My Story. I'm now declaring our year of CaringBridge complete. It's time to move on, and I'm ready.

Tonight at chorus rehearsal I completed the year with my chorus director, saying that some of my best memories are about the times when the chorus invited me up, on crutches or wheelchair or scooter, to sing a song, or at times for them to sing "You'll Never Walk Alone."

And that's how I've always felt here, too – with you, I never walked alone. You made such a difference for me, at a time when that made all the difference in my experience. Please really deeply get my acknowledgement for the difference you made in my life. I may still have occasion to post here rarely, but for the most part I'm done.

What's next? Take it out into the world. I invite you to join the e-patient movement. Follow their blogs, follow my new blog, contribute your own stories and opinions. Read their manifesto. Tell other people about it – it's all about what we (you) did here!

As I write this, since the start it's been: 365 days, 15,227 visits, 204 journal posts, 1,061 guestbook messages ... and one wonderful, amazing, totally transformational year. In several ways, I owe my life to you. Thank you all so very, very much for your support ... now go have a great rest of your life!

Chapter 16: In Search of a New Life

September 25 – December 17, 2007

After my final Interleukin treatment in August 2007, it became clear that I had won my battle against cancer, at least for the time being. I found I'd been given a "free replay"on life: my mets had shrunk, my CAT scan was relatively clean, the burden of the extra house was gone. So what was I going to do with my new life?

My thoughts took shape by fits and starts during the next six months – only vaguely at first, and then (with my discovery of the e-patient movement) with sudden clarity. Everything fell into place: high tech, social change, communities – and a healthcare system searching for its bearings. The following posts chronicle how my thinking evolved.

Tuesday, September 25, 2007 11:02 PM

Early detection

As you know, I've been wondering what I'm going to create as a future, to make use of this experience. Increasingly, it seems clear to me that it's going to be about early detection. I figure my January shoulder x-ray gave me a six-week head start, because it was six weeks later that my thigh started hurting like hell.

By 2/26 they'd done the bone scan and found the huge met there. So even without the shoulder x-ray we would have known by then. But, see, because of the earlier detection, my nephrectomy was already scheduled for March 6. And the nephrectomy needed to be done before starting the IL-2, to reduce the total tumor burden.

Remember the strange growth that appeared on my tongue just before I started on IL-2? As I said earlier, we'll never know what that was, but I strongly suspect it was a metastasis, growing out of my tongue muscle. What if I hadn't been ready for IL-2 when that thing emerged? If it had grown there for weeks while I waited to start treatment?

So do I think early detection is a big deal? You bet I do.

Remember that the American Cancer Society's big thing for the coming year is that all the science that's gone before us will do no good if people don't have the insurance to pay for early detection.

I request that you take responsibility for spreading this discussion, when the chance arises: I'm sure a lot of people out there haven't heard the American Cancer Society's message. They have a very good record of changing our global conversations to create change – here's your chance to honor THIS community by being part of that change. Tell people.

Randy Pausch

In case you haven't heard, this Carnegie Mellon professor was on Good Morning America. Your homework: learn what you can about him.

He was dying of pancreatic cancer and was being phenomenal about it; much of "who he was being" about it bears strong resemblance to our story here. He says "We cannot change the cards we're dealt, only the way we play them."

I was a little irritated that the GMA interviewers were so incredulous about his attitude that they almost seemed to be saying "Why aren't you crying for me??"

But that's just me, complaining – no power in that. See the actual footage.

As the article says, he realized that he had the opportunity to create "The Last Lecture." He delivered it the following week – it's about living life to the fullest. A video of the entire hour-plus is available online. (To see it, go to YouTube and search for "The last lecture.")

He is inspiring. As I say, learn what you can about him – he's all over if you Google him.

Laugh, Sing, and Eat Like a Pig

Thursday, October 18, 2007 12:40 AM

Tonight was the Beth Israel Deaconess board dinner. It was quite an event: dozens of seriously high-level medicos and trustee-level people who had spent the day shadowing one employee or another in their jobs, to see what it's like on the front lines. I chatted with several of them at the reception, and was very pleased with how open they were. My experience was that they were truly interested in what I thought.

Before dessert we had a panel discussion about patient experiences. I had the great joy (really) of sitting next to the phenomenal author Monique Doyle Spencer, who is every bit as much of a punk as when she wrote *The Courage Muscle*. The other panelist was a guy who'd had some horrifying experiences as a patient, 10 years ago, before the turnaround that took place 5-6 years ago, and problems since then.

This openness and candor is characteristic of the BIDMC culture – at least the part that I've seen. It's present constantly in Paul Levy's blog. Here they are, one of the best hospitals at patient satisfaction, and they're striving for more, starting with listening to people at the receiving end. And what we had tonight was about 50 dedicated people, in the middle of a two-day training session, avidly listening to those people.

At least 20 of them came up to us personally at the end, looking like they'd been moved by the experience. Several said "We learned a lot from our shadowing today, and your words tonight made it real for us." I think they really were moved.

I had the sense that we tonight were on the leading edge of transforming how healthcare is delivered. To be sure, things are not perfect – but these people are actively engaged in doing something about it, starting by talking to us on the receiving end. And LISTENING to what they heard in response. Huzzah!

Well, folks, I told them they should have something like CaringBridge built right into their website. Because YOU have made such a difference in my experience. [The following year the hospital did begin to offer a service like CaringBridge, built into their website. They listened!]

174

Friday, December 7, 2007

What's it gonna take?

What's it gonna take to be so present that I reliably do what I said I was gonna do?

I say I'm going to practice singing, then I do something else. Three days later I say I'm going to pay my bills, then I do something else.

The point isn't that I'm being "bad" when this happens. It's not that I "should" pay my bills that day, or sing that day. The point is that I said I was going to, and I meant it – so what the heck happened?? It's as if I turned on my blinker, turned the steering wheel, and nothing happened.

Well, actually something happened – I went straight, maybe I hit something, and I certainly didn't go where I said I was going. In any case it wasn't what I said would happen, and not what I put effort into. Isn't that weird??

So what's it going to take to be fully alert, present, and "connected to my wheels" so I'm actually the one who says how my life is going?

The irony of this, of course, is that I've spent the past year SAYING how my life is going to go, and succeeding. Nothing could stop me, because everything was at stake. I was, quite literally, living as if my life depended on it.

This reminds me of something from the "est" training (precursor to Landmark): "A game is what you have when what's not so, is more important than what is so." A current example might be CalvinBall, where Calvin & Hobbes make up rules on the fly – none of it is real, it's all an agreement about what's important. (Of course, they supposedly know it's all made up, because they change the rules whenever they want, and it goes the way they say. The problem comes when you're not aware of the game.)

And est continued: "When what is so becomes more important, the game is over." Like, Calvin & Hobbes are just there, standing at what used to be the goal line. Except now they're just present.

I'd say, when you know what you want but you're not getting there, it's a pretty sure sign that you're playing CalvinBall and you don't know it.

I want to get back to where I was when I was sick. Isn't that weird? But – and I'm not making this up – as I wrote this post, in the background there was an episode of the TV show "House," about a cranky doctor, and in it, a character was ticked off because his diagnosis of terminal cancer turned out to be false. "I've never been as present and alive as I was these past few months – and now you took that away from me." Yeah well, you and I know nobody took anything away from him – it's all in his mind. Mine too.

So the question is, what's it gonna take, to be that present all the time, so I actually do what I say? I know from recent experience that I get a lot of joy when it goes the way I said.

Friday, December 7, 2007 11:07 PM

Just this week I've been reflecting on the fact that I am NOT as fully alive as I was, when my life was at stake. I'm not happy about that. I find myself back in the world of "I can't because I have these other obligations." And I say that despite knowing full well that it's all made up, all imaginary "have to" stuff.

That's not to say I've lost the ability to experience joy. I love singing more than ever, and I love my work (though I wish I were faster at it), and I have more love in my relationships than ever before. I even find myself on the verge of telling some people I love them, just in the moment, without having the sort of prior relationship that would make that "appropriate."

But despite all that, the moments of my life no longer feel like "This is it – there ain't nowhere to get to, this is IT. NOW." Also this week, tightly intertwined with that, I realized what I'm going to do with the new blog. Landmark people occasionally talk about "living as if your life depended on it" – living every moment as if your whole life depended on what you were doing right now. You can bet that's how I lived this year – but here I am back to "Can't do that now, because I have to xyz." What I'm going to do

176

with the new blog is inquire into "living as if your life depended on it."

♦   ♦   ♦

Meanwhile, on a much more mundane front: as my annual physical approaches (mid-January) I'm watching my weight, and I must say, I don't like seeing that my weight started dropping, as it was doing a year ago. Clearly, part of me is worried that it might be cancer waking up again. SO, I look forward to Monday afternoon's results meeting with the oncology team – the first one in 3 months, if you can believe that! Once I have evidence that the cancer's stable or gone, I'll be confident that it's safe to lose weight. :-)

I WOULD LIKE TO HAVE THE "IT KEEPS ME ALIVE" PART WITHOUT BEING ON THE EDGE OF DEATH!

Monday, December 17, 2007 12:22 AM

Regarding my new blog, something's happening that feels odd. When I started it a few weeks ago, I'd had this burst of clarity that it was going to be about what I'm doing with my new life. But now it seems like I'm over that – like, yeah, that's in the past, but even the "new life" part is done now. Sorta like we broke the sound barrier, and it sure was dramatic and bumpy, and now here we are on the other side.

Anyway, I'm continuing to tell people about declaring it complete as of the end of this month. Had the first part of that conversation at work this week, and will continue Monday.

Chapter 17: Patient Dave becomes e-Patient Dave

January 23 – January 28, 2008

Wednesday, January 23, 2008 5:14 PM

Heads up!

Holy crap, look at this: The eDocAmerica blog (edocamerica. blogspot.com). Then look at his other posts about "e-Patients." "e-Patients are those that use email and the internet to become empowered to manage their own health and become partners with their providers. From saving lives to saving dollars, this blog both entertains and instructs in ways to use the internet for better healthcare. Approach with caution – this may radically change your views about your approach to the healthcare system!" WOOT!, as my daughter says. More on this in the next few days, my babies. Stuff is in the wind.

Thursday, January 24, 2008 11:37 PM

E-PATIENT SCHOLARS WORKING GROUP

The other night I said I'd learned of this group, and the concept of e-patients, who educate themselves and do research to become more effective partners with their patients. And I said stuff is in the wind.

Here's the news, folks. I've been invited to go join this small group at a retreat they're having at the end of February. Part of me is thrilled beyond belief that I'd get to spend time with this incredible list of people. Another part of me sees this as a humbling and wonderful challenge to educate myself and make the best use of the opportunity, both to learn and to share my experiences and perspectives.

Looks like a fine answer to my question about "What am I going to make of this past year's experience?" Homework: reading as much as I can of the e-Patients Manifesto (www.acor.org/e-patients-wiki). It's both a PDF (to download) and a living Wiki – a document that can be (and is) edited by the community of those who need and use it.

Friday, January 25, 2008 8:09 PM

This e-patients group is a wonderful thing. I'm feeling turbo-charged. If you're into empowerment or any form of "power to the people" or "let me do it myself, thank you" or personal responsibility, this is something you want to learn about.

It's not just about cancer, it's about taking personal responsibility for managing your own health.

What a wonderful web site: e-patients.net has a "quote-a-matic" thing that dispenses wisdom like fortune cookies. A couple of quickies I noticed:

> It is not the strongest that survive, nor the more intelligent, but those most responsive to change.
> – Charles Darwin

> The future is here; it's just not evenly distributed yet.
> – William Gibson

> External pressure will be necessary to move the system toward meaningful change.
> – Don Berwick

There are also a host of useful links about the e-patient movement. Example: a NYTimes blog post about "Medical Googlers" and why doctors should work with them, not reject them. HUZZAH!

One member of the group is Gilles Frydman, who founded all of ACOR. And I'm going to get to meet him and do the weekend retreat with him. Huzzah. Will WE have things to talk about.

Sooooo, everybody, see what you started when you helped me stay alive??? Thank you yet again.

Monday, January 28, 2008

e-Patient? Yes, e-Patient.

In the past few days, with my discovery on 1/23 of the e-Patient Scholars Working Group, my entire outlook on life has changed – so much so that I'm changing the title of this blog from "Patient Dave" to "e-Patient Dave."

That's because I've found my purpose for this blog. And that in turn is because my experience over the past year is a ridiculously close match for the principles and practices recommended by the group. So I think I've found the answer to a question I've asked in recent months: "What am I going to do, what am I going to create in the world, out of my experiences of the past year?"

I'd heard about this "movement" (my term, not theirs) earlier in the month from Dr. Danny Sands, my primary physician, a member of the group.

It's been a busy few days for me. As I've said to several friends, "It's as if I've discovered a parallel universe where everyone speaks a language I thought nobody else spoke."

I can't believe I went through last year without knowing about this group. Well, I do now.

Monday, January 28, 2008 10:20 AM

How fun is THIS?? I forwarded my post about my blog change to Dr. Sands, and he passed it to the e-Patients group, and today I'm on their blog!

Ginny just said "Perhaps there's a reason you got sick." I personally am not in favor of cancer as a means to ANYTHING, but it occurred to me – yeah, if life hands you lemons, why not make lemonade – for everyone?

See, it's a lesson we learned together .... let's share it far and wide, everyone.

YAYYYYYYYYYYYYYYYY!!!!!!

Epilog: A blogger, "just a patient," bends the course of national policy

April 1 – June 6, 2009

In the spring of 2009 I blogged about my experience with health data systems, such as those offered by Google (Google Health) and Microsoft (HealthVault). Unexpectedly, I found myself caught up in a media and blog firestorm that led to being involved in policy discussions in Washington and, ultimately, to leaving my old career and going into health advocacy full time. This chapter contains those posts.

It was a remarkable period, and it made me realize how important the voice of the patient can be in the rapidly shifting landscape of health data systems. It also made me realize that non-medical people have much to offer as healthcare comes online – because IT outside healthcare is way, way ahead of health IT.

Today I know a lot more about PHRs, health IT, and EMRs (electronic medical record systems), so if I were to start reporting it now I'd say it in a more nuanced way. But that makes what happened more remarkable: a blogger sitting in his living room in Nashua, NH, with no expertise specific to health IT, writes a post that stops a policy initiative in its tracks. So these posts are reproduced here as originally posted (with a limited amount of editing by my publisher), as events unfolded, without benefit of hindsight.

Tuesday, May 20, 2008

The launch of Google Health

There's a lot of talk this week about the launch of Google Health. As much as I love everything online, I have grave concerns about this. I wrote about it earlier, speaking on general principle. But now that the thing is finally launched, the full terms of service are out (the fine print), and my concerns are even greater.

#1 on my list is that due to some legalese (Google itself isn't a healthcare provider), Google Health is not subject to HIPAA privacy regulations. Google isn't required to observe HIPAA protections to keep your data private, and there are no legal consequences if they don't.

Of greater concern is that the whole point of Google Health is that they send your information to others you select, at which point the data is completely out of Google's control.

And that doesn't begin to get into the sociological/political concerns I raised in January – questions of what to do when Google says "Really, just trust us" in the absence of any policing.

Let's hope it turns out there's actually no privacy concern. Then all we'd have to worry about is whether to trust Google in the first place.

Sunday, February 22, 2009

I'm putting my data in Google and HealthVault

I've decided to go ahead and put my data in Google Health and MicroSoft HealthVault.

(Note: MicroSoft HealthVault is a different kind of thing from Google Health. About the only thing they have in common is that I can put my health data in them. For this post I'll only discuss Google, but the concerns people have about the two are similar, and so are my thoughts.)

This is something of an earthquake on The Dave Planet. When Google Health was first announced in January 2008, I was completely distrustful and wrote: "GOOG's stock is doing great and I love their free tools, but there's no way in hell I'm giving them sensitive personal data, regardless of what their policy says. New motto for 2008: Don't Be Stupid."

It was a direct slam against Google's long-professed unofficial motto "Don't Be Evil." I expressed my concern that Google might succumb to government pressure and dish out personal medical information that someone had entrusted to Google Health. I cited how Google had caved in to China's government, and how Google CEO Eric Schmidt had severely punished CNET.com for Googling his personal information and publishing it. I saw hypocrisy.

Others agreed. One online forum discussed the potential for abuse, given that Google collects enormous information about each of us as we browse the web and use Google's search features – they know what you've searched for and (through ordinary marketing software that most websites install) they know what sites you've visited.

They say they won't use that info; but... what if? What if an evil politician (take your pick: Dick Cheney, Hillary Clinton, Putin) puts the squeeze on Google to disclose such information so they can use it against you? That's less improbable than what actually did happen to Valerie Plame. In cases like that, laws will not protect you.

In online discussion groups, experts in "search engine marketing" joked about it: If Google knows you have a kidney problem, then the Google Maps "Street View" feature might point out potential kidney donors, and the ads on the side of your screen might start promoting bathtubs and ice. (Yes, people did joke about that.)

That's a bit over the top, but you get the point.

Similar concerns continue today – this delightful image appeared on a ZDNet post this month, titled "Is Google Health corrupt?"

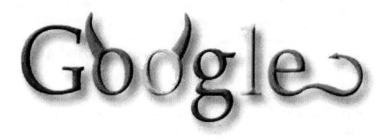

So why have I gone over?

First, in the past year an increasingly wide range of people I trust have said "The data you're concerned about is already not as secure as you think." That doesn't leave me any more comfortable but I've come to accept that my choice of action won't make much difference.

Second, and more importantly, I'm concluding that we can do more good by aggregating our data into large, anonymized databanks that smart software can analyze to look for patterns. Early detection means early intervention means fewer crises.

Diabetics are already starting to do things like this. And the Cambridge, MA-based PatientsLikeMe.com is a full-blown example of a community (ALS/Lou Gehrig's disease) where patients are tired of waiting for the medical industry to produce results. They're uploading their data (anonymized), sharing it, looking for patterns, even creating their own clinical trials.

The third aspect, ultimately the deciding one, is something I see all the time in my day job, where we study new software tools: the power of "mash-ups." That's the ability to slap together two pieces of software (or data) that were created without knowing that the other one exists, and making something new out of them without anyone planning it in advance. Things can just grow in any direction people want.

Mash-ups are a big part of what makes the Web what it is today: Anyone can put a Yahoo Map on their web site, I can take someone's YouTube video and put it on my blog, etc.

The power happens because this lets people create software gadgets without knowing how they'll be used, it lets people build tools that use data without knowing where the data will come from, and it lets people build big new systems just by assembling them out of "software Legos."

And in healthcare, that's what free public tools like Google Health and Microsoft HealthVault enable. Here's the personal example that hit me recently and tipped me:

When I was discharged from the hospital after my first week of Interleukin, I was given a complex medication schedule grid –

which had to be created with pencil and ruler by a highly trained nurse.

This was not a sensible use of her time. So, being a software thinker, I spec'd out a "Med Minder" program that would take prescription instructions ("take this one 3x/day, take this one with meals," etc.) and spit out a nicely printed daily schedule. I had additional ideas: "mash it up" with a database of pill images so you can see what pills to take; "mash it up" with a database of different Walgreen's pillboxes so you can see what to put in each cell of your particular pillbox.

I talked to a few people about it and hadn't found anyone interested in the idea.

But at the Google Health booth at a recent trade show, look what I saw: software that takes your prescription info from Google Health and tells you how to fill your pillbox.

It was an epiphany: put my data in there, and I get access to mash-ups. All kinds of potential tools that I know could be useful become possible. The healthcare establishment isn't getting around to doing them, but ordinary data geeks are.

So here's how it boils down: My goal is to help create a new world where healthcare is enormously more efficient than it is today, and where important new developments happen enormously faster than they do today. And with that in mind, the advantages of uploading our data far outweigh the risks.

So I'm in.

◆   ◆   ◆

When I clicked the button to export my data, Google displayed many things that weren't true. It puzzled me. I discussed it with members of the e-patients working group, and we realized that Google was correctly showing what the hospital had sent.

It took several weeks to think out what could be said on our blog that would do any good. The cheap, cheesy thing for a blogger to do would be to toss out insults, but there's no use in that. The useful question was what could be said that would be of value to e-patients.

Laugh, Sing, and Eat Like a Pig

I dropped a preliminary note on March 18, asking people to think, and two weeks later wrote the full story.

Wednesday, April 1, 2009

Imagine someone had been managing your data, and then you looked.

This is a complex post, so don't jump to any conclusions.

Two weeks ago (gad, was it that long?) I asked you to think about something for a few days:

> Imagine that for all your life, and your parents' lives, your money had been managed by other people who had extensive training and licensing. Imagine that all your records were in their possession, and you could occasionally see parts of them, but you just figured the pros had it under control.

> Imagine that you knew you weren't a financial planner but you wanted to take as much responsibility as you could – to participate. Imagine that some money managers (not all, but many) attacked people who wanted to make their own decisions, saying "Who's the financial planner here?"

> Then imagine that one day you were allowed to see the records, and you found out there were a whole lot of errors, and the people carefully guarding your data were not as on top of things as everyone thought.

Two weeks before that post, I'd had a personal breakthough in my thinking. For a year I'd been a rabid enemy of Google Health, but now I said I would put my data in Google and HealthVault: "I'm concluding that we can do more good by aggregating our data into large, anonymized databanks that smart software can analyze to look for patterns. Early detection means early intervention means fewer crises."

And I observed that the power of Web 2.0 "mash-ups" …

> …lets people create software gadgets without knowing how they'll be used, it lets people build tools that use data

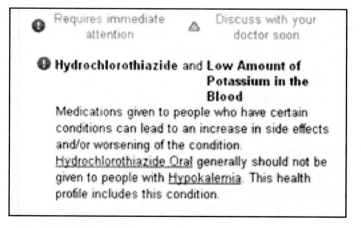

When I loaded my health data into Google, it gave me a dire-sounding alert: "Requires immediate attention".

without knowing where the data will come from, and it lets people build big new systems just by assembling them out of "software Legos."

So, I said, "I'm in." I decided to punch the big red button and copy my personal health data into Google Health.

I've discussed what follows with hospital staff; this isn't gossip behind anyone's back. IMO, empowered people don't gossip, they communicate clearly and directly with the people involved.

Having decided to upload my data, I went into my hospital's patient portal and clicked the button to do it. I checked the boxes for all the options and clicked Upload. It was pretty quick.

But WTF? An alarm: "! Requires immediate attention"

Okay, yes, hydrochlorothiazide is my blood pressure medication.

But low potassium? That was true when I was hospitalized two years ago, not now. What's going on?

Then I saw the list of "conditions" it told Google I have. Here's a partial screen grab:

Profile summary 🖶Print▼

Conditions

Acidosis More info »

Anxiety Disorder More info »

Aortic Aneurysm

Arthroplasty - Hip, Total Replacement

Bone Disease

CANCER

Cancer Metastasis to Bone

This is part of the list of conditions Google Health said I had.

And here's the complete list: (spoiler alert; this stuff is biological)

Acidosis

Anxiety Disorder

Aortic Aneurysm

Arthroplasty - Hip, Total Replacemt

Bone Disease

CANCER

Cancer Metastasis to Bone

Cardiac Impairment

CHEST MASS

Chronic Lung Disease

Depressed Mood

DEPRESSION

Diarrhea

Elevated Blood Pressure

Hair Follicle Inflammation w Abscess in Sweat Gland Areas

HEALTH MAINTENANCE

HYDRADENITIS

HYPERTENSION

Intestinal Parasitic Infection

Kidney Problems Causing a Decreased Amount of Urine to be Passed

Lightheaded

Low Amount of Calcium in the Blood

Low Amount of Potassium in the Blood

Malignant Neoplastic Disease
Migraine Headache
MIGRAINES
Nausea and Vomiting Nephrosis
PSYCH
Rash
Spread of Cancer to Brain or Spinal Cord
Swollen Lymph Nodes

Yes, ladies and germs, everything I've ever had was listed. With almost no dates attached. It did have the correct date for my very first visit, and for Chest Mass, the x-ray that first found the undiagnosed lesion. But the date for CANCER, the big one, was 5/25/07 – four months after the diagnosis. And no other line item had any date. For instance, the "anxiety" diagnosis was when I was puking my guts out during my cancer treatment. I got medicated for that, justified by the intelligent observation (diagnosis) that I was anxious. But you wouldn't know that from looking at this.

See how some of the listed conditions have links for More Info? Let's see, I was diagnosed with optical migraine, an odd symptom that produces a little dazzling pattern in one eye occasionally. (It happened for a brief period and stopped. I diagnosed myself, actually, by researching my symptoms and linking to a site with illustrations that matched what I was seeing. (That's what e-patients do; it saves time in the doctor's office.) But optical migraine is not the impression you'd get from reading my conditions list – in fact during my cancer workup one resident said "But you have headaches, right?" "No," I said – "optical migraines, but without pain."

So for that item in the conditions list, I clicked More Info. I didn't get more info (i.e. accurate info) about my diagnosis, just Google's encyclopedia-style article about migraines in general. (An optical migraine has little in common with migraines in general.)

The really fun stuff, though, is that some of the conditions transmitted are things I've never had: aortic aneurysm and metastases to the brain or spine.

So what the heck??

◆　　◆　　◆

I've been discussing this with the docs in the back room here on the e-patient blog, and they quickly figured out what was going on before I confirmed it: they sent insurance billing codes into Google Health, not doctors' diagnoses. And as those in the know are well aware, in our system today, insurance billing codes may bear no resemblance to reality.

(I don't want to get into the whole thing right now, but basically if a doc needs to bill insurance for something and the list of billing codes doesn't happen to include exactly what your condition is, they cram it into something else so the stupid system will accept it. And, btw, everyone in the business is apparently accustomed to the system being stupid, so it's no surprise that nobody can tell whether things are making any sense: nobody counts on the data to be meaningful in the first place.)

We could (and will someday) have a nice big discussion about why the hell the most expensive healthcare system in the world (America's) STILL doesn't have an accurate data model, but that's not my point. We'll get to that.

◆　　◆　　◆

And now we get to why I said, at the outset, don't jump to conclusions. My personal experience with medical records transfer, by itself, wouldn't justify staying up to 3 in the morning writing a 3700-word post. The BIG question is, do you know what's in your medical record? And THAT is a question worth answering. For every one of you.

See, every time I speak at a conference I point out that my 12/6/2003 x-ray identified me as a 53-year-old woman. I admit I have the man-boob thing going on, but not THAT much. And here's the next thing: it took me months to get that error corrected, because nobody's in the habit of actually fixing errors.

Think about THAT. I mean, some EMR (electronic medical records) pontificators are saying "Online data in the hospital won't do any good at the scene of a car crash" because your data's not there at the crash. Well, GOOD: you think I'd want the EMTs to think I have an aneurysm, anxiety, migraines and brain mets?? Yet if I hadn't punched that button, I never would have known my data in the system might be erroneous.

And this isn't just academic: in Minnesota a while back, a patient's good kidney was removed and the cancerous one was left in place, which arose at least partly out of an error that ended up in the hospital's electronic medical records system. Their patient portal allowed patients and family to view some radiology reports, but not the one that contained the fateful error.

◆   ◆   ◆

But my problems with Google Health weren't limited to just the erroneous information. The kicker came when I got over my surprise about what had been transferred, and realized what had not: my history. Weight, BP, and lab data were all still in the portal, and not in Google Health.

So I went back and looked at the boxes I'd checked for what data to send, and son of a gun, there were only three boxes: diagnoses, medications, and allergies. Nothing about lab data, nothing about vital signs.

And of the three things it did transmit:

- What was transferred as diagnoses was actually billing codes.

- The one item of medication data that made it across was correct, but it was only my current BP med. (Which, btw, Google Health said had an urgent conflict with my two-years-ago potassium condition, which had been sent without a date). It sent no medication history, not even the fact that I'd had four weeks of high dosage Interleukin-2, which just MIGHT be useful to have in my personal health record, eh?

- The allergies data did NOT include the one thing I must not ever, ever violate: no steroids (e.g. cortisone) ever again (they suppress the immune system), because it'll interfere with the immune treatment that saved my life and is still active within me. (I am well, but my type of cancer normally recurs.)

In other words, the data that arrived in Google Health was essentially unusable.

In any case, my hospital is very proactive and empowering to staff about root cause analysis for failures, and they'll add any process or form that can catch potential errors. That, at least, is good.

◆　◆　◆

I work with data in my day job. (I do marketing analytics for a software company. We import and export data all the time.) I understand what it takes to make sure you've got clean data, and make sure the data models line up on both sides of a transfer. I know what it's like to look at a transfer gone bad, and hunt down where the errors arose, so they don't happen again. And I'm fairly good at sniffing out how something went wobbly.

And you know what I suspect? I suspect processes for data integrity in healthcare are largely absent, by ordinary business standards. I suspect there are few, if any, processes in place to prevent wrong data from entering the system, or tracking down the cause when things do go awry.

And here's the real kicker: my hospital is one of the more advanced in the US in the use of electronic medical records. So I suspect that most healthcare institutions don't even know what it means to have processes in place to ensure that data doesn't get screwed up in the system, or if it does, to trace how it happened.

Consider the article in *Fast Company* in late 2008 about an innovative program at Geisinger. Anecdotally, it ended with this chiller:

> … a list of everybody that accessed the medical record
> from the time he was seen in the clinic to two weeks post-
> op. There were 113 people listed – and every one had an
> appropriate reason to be in that chart. It shocked all of us.
> We all knew this was a team sport, but to recognize it was
> that big a team, every one of whom is empowered to screw
> it up – that makes me toss and turn in my sleep.

In my day job, the sales and marketing system we use (Salesforce. com) has very granular authorizations for who can change what, and we can switch on a feature (at no extra cost) to track every change that's made on any data field. Why? Because in some business situations it's important to know where errors arose – an error might cause business damage, or an employee might sue over a missed quota.

So I'm thinking, why on earth don't medical records systems have these protections? If a popular-priced sales management system has audit traces, to prevent an occasional lawsuit over a sales rep's missed commission, why isn't this a standard feature in high-priced medical records systems?

In any case, in the several weeks since these discoveries started, as far as I know they haven't figured out how my wrong data got in there. And without knowing how the wrong data got in, there's not a prayer of identifying what process failed.

♦   ♦   ♦

BUT AS I SAID, this is not about my hospital. Nor is this a slam on Google Health. (And I haven't even touched HealthVault.) None of that is my point.

Rather, my point is about the data that was already in my PHR, uninspected. For that, let's return to my previous post:

> Then imagine that one day you were allowed to see the records, and you found out there were a whole lot of errors, and the people carefully guarding your data were not as on top of things as everyone thought.

In my day job, when we discover that a data set has not been well managed, we have to make a decision: do we go back and clean up the data (which takes time and money), or do we decide to just start "living clean" from now on?

My point, my advice to e-patients, is: Find out what's in your medical record. What's in your wallet, medically speaking? Better find out, and correct what's wrong.

Get started, manually, moving your data into Google Health, HealthVault, or some such system. I've heard there are similar PHR systems (personal health records), not free but modestly priced, that can reportedly make this easier. Let's start working, now, on a reliable interoperable data model.

I know the policy wonks are going to scream "Not possible!" and I know there are lots of good reasons why it's impossibly complex. But y'know what else? I've talked to enough e-patients to be confident that we patients want working, interoperable data. And if you-all in the vendor community can't work it out, we will start growing one. It won't be as sophisticated as yours, but as with all disruptive technologies , it will be what we want. And we'll add features to ours, faster than you can hold meetings to discuss us.

I have to say, while researching this post I was quite surprised at how very, very far the industry has to go before reaching a viable universal data model. New standards are in development, but I'm certain that it will take years and years and gazillions of dollars before any of that is a reality. (What, like costs aren't high enough already?) In the meantime, your data is probably not going to flow very easily from system to system. Far, far harder than (for instance) downloading your data to Quicken from different credit card companies and banks.

Let's start working, now, on an open source EMR/PHR system. The open source community creates functionality faster, and more bug-free, than commercial vendors do – and nobody can latch onto proprietary data in such systems to milk more margin out of us... because it ain't proprietary.

The great limitation of open source is that it's generally not well funded. But you know what? Every person in America (including the software engineers) is motivated to have good reliable healthcare systems, and I assert that the industry ain't getting' it done on their own. It's fine with me if industry vendors come along too – but I would not stake my life on their moving fast enough for my needs. Or your mother's.

Want a case study with real consequences? Recall what happened last year to famed Linux guru Doc Searls when he couldn't read his own scan data, because good cross-platform image viewing tools weren't available. Doc was mobilized by his own experience with a procedure called an ERCP (Endoscopic Retrograde Cholangiopancreatography), which had a "1 in 20 chance" of causing pancreatitis. Doc proved to be a one in twenty, and after battling pancreatitis learned that the MRI that led to the ERCP was misinterpreted, the procedure was unnecessary, that he had stumbled into a system that is "built to treat templates, not the pile of combined oddities and typicalities that comprise a sixty-year-old human being." (His prescription: the patient should be the platform and "the point of integration." Your records should travel with you and be under your control; they shouldn't stay with a given hospital or physician that you visited.)

Well, okay, so Doc was a year ahead of me. I'm catching on. This illustrates why I think people from outside the profession may be our greatest asset in building what patients really need: patients tend to build what they want. And we who work with data all day know that these problems are not unsolvable.

◆ ◆ ◆

My bottom line: I think we ought to get our data into secure online systems, and we shouldn't expect it to happen with the push of a button. It'll take work. So let's get to work.

You know the work will be good for you, and heaven only knows what you'll learn in the process. You'll certainly end up more aware of your health data than when you started. And that's a good thing.

◆ ◆ ◆

I was completely unprepared for what happened next. Scores of comments appeared on the post, including many from people I'd never heard of. Eventually I learned that I'd unwittingly stepped into the middle of a big Washington policy issue: many people were proposing that insurance records should be used as our actual medical records.

It took a month to catch my breath. In mid-May I summarized the previous seven weeks.

Laugh, Sing, and Eat Like a Pig

Tuesday, May 19, 2009 8:08 PM

I'm starting to catch my breath after what's been a completely wild seven weeks. On the night of March 31 I started writing about what happened when I tried to move my health records out of my hospital's system and into Google Health.

The post drew a lot of response from people in the blogosphere, but not the general public, and no interest at all from the hospital initially.

Then I got a call from the Boston *Globe* saying that they felt the story was important. They took ten days to do a very carefully researched and written story that hit on April 13: "Electronic Health Records Raise Doubt." It was on the front page of the Globe, and on the inside was a photo they'd taken, which made me look like I wanted to kill someone. :) All hell broke loose.

That very day the hospital's CIO (chief information officer) wrote on his blog that they would promptly meet with my doctor and me, and the product manager of Google Health, to discuss the mess. Two nights later that call happened, and we all agreed that transmitting billing codes was not sensible, so Google decided to stop accepting them and the hospital agreed to stop transmitting them.

I was a little irked that they still didn't want to say it was simply a mistake – they wanted to say that billing codes could be "confusing." Well, when the thing says I had a stroke, and I didn't, that's not confusing, it's wrong. In the end the hospital published a statement saying (correctly!) that it was a mistake to do it. Good for them!

Once it was in the *Globe* (which covers a lot of health issues because of all the Boston hospitals) it went all over the place. It was stressful for me because a lot of idiots on blogs and in other media only read the *Globe* article (not my post) and misinterpreted it, which bugged me because I'd worked hard to be careful in what I did and didn't say. I also got calls and emails from all over creation, which took lots of time, as I tried to make sure everyone got the story straight.

196

As fate would have it, the following week (April 21-22) there was a big health conference in Boston, where my doctor and I were already slated to speak. By that time the story was all over the place, because of two related things: (1) the federal stimulus package includes $19 billion for incentives for docs to start using EMRs (electronic medical records), and (2) a lot of people have figured that to get the systems started up, they would just grab everyone's billing records and move them into the EMRs. Well, not any more they don't think that.

At one point on the first day of the conference the conference manager asked if I was there to make comments. I happened to be up in the balcony of the ballroom, and I stood up and spoke. Everyone turned and looked up. To me it was nothing, but people who've been going to medical conferences for years said it was a profound moment: medical experts turning and (literally) looking up to a patient.

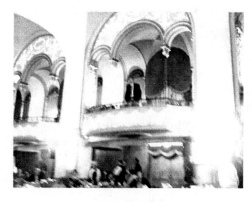

Who says doctors don't look up to e-patients?I happened to be sitting in the ballroom's balcony when I was called on, which had an amusing effect when I spoke. A cell phone catured this picutre.

Photo courtesy of Linda Davis, via Ted Eytan's blog.

One person on Twitter said I looked like the Pope. :) (I hope you know I'm not getting a big head about this – it's fun but as the saying goes, "I'm still just Dad, to my daughter." And my boss still says "Where's that report??")

That day Forbes.com called about the story, too; their piece ran that Friday.

The next day I was slated to speak, and I took this moment of people's attention to broadcast the message of Participatory Medicine, in which patients play an active role in their care.

There was another *Globe* article, a *Globe* editorial, more posts on my blog, a very good article on the Information Quality Trainwrecks blog, and much more.

◆　　◆　　◆

That was a fortuitous conference, following fortuitously on the Google Health story, because a bunch of press and government people were there. As a result, I was invited to Washington to participate in a think-tank session at the Center for Democracy and Technology, which has been tasked by the FTC and the Dept of Health & Human Services (HHS) with contributing thoughts on electronic medical records.

I didn't talk about the problems that had happened – that's all in the past. I talked about the good that can come from people having access to their records. And I spoke, with passion, that one of the most fundamental human rights must be the right of a desperate person to try to save themselves, and if that includes being able to take your records and go somewhere that has an additional treatment, so be it.

See, today's privacy regulations are too often misinterpreted in ways that make it difficult for us to even see our own records, never mind take the data somewhere else. The regulations have been so tortured that in one case, a woman discovered that someone else's records had been mixed in with hers, and the privacy goons promptly (and incorrectly) locked her out of her own records – because they contained some data that she wasn't entitled to see!

I could go on and on, but you get the picture.

It's funny, because all this started out with my just trying to move my data into Google Health, but it's turned into something of a spotlight, in which I'm talking about participatory medicine.

So let me ask you: do YOU know what's in YOUR medical record? A day might come when you need that data to be correct. As one well-known doc said in the original Globe article, if you were wheeled into an emergency room with wrong data in your record, they could be steered away from a life-saving treatment, or they could be steered TO a treatment that could kill you.

Medicine is 10-20 years behind most of the world in getting good reliable online data. We'll get there, and you can help.

Saturday, June 6, 2009

Last Tuesday, June 2, I was on a consumer panel at a board meeting of the National eHealth Collaborative. This is a heady group to be addressing; nine of these people are on the advisory committees that are working directly with David Blumenthal, Obama's National Coordinator for Health IT, to set policy and standards.

The topic was whether "consumer pull" would encourage health-care providers to adopt electronic medical record systems (EMRs). (Like, if you and I keep asking our doctors and hospitals to let us see our data online, will they be more likely to get off their butts and GET our data online??)

All I can say is, if I have anything to do with it, consumers (that's you) will be clamoring to see their medical records, both to check their accuracy and for the reason I sent my data to Google Health in the first place: to get involved in their care, to be responsible, to participate.

Go thou into the wilderness and clamor for access!

Appendix A
e-Patient White Paper: Chapter Summaries

In 2008 I began to educate myself about the e-patient movement. In mid-summer I realized several things about the e-Patient White Paper: it was full of transformational insights, it was too long for a popular document, and parts of it just weren't sinking in.

So I took on the task of teaching it to others, by writing chapter summaries. I posted them on my blog, and the e-patient group decided to add them to the online wiki edition of the white paper. Here they are, just as I posted them – including the less-than-formal "wow" on the opening quote. :-)

The e-Patient White Paper was published in 2007 by the e-Patient Scholars Working Group, completing the life work of Dr. Tom Ferguson. It begins with this quote:

> "[People] are suddenly nomadic gatherers of knowledge...
> informed as never before...
> involved in the social process as never before...
> [as] we extend our central nervous system globally..."
>
> – Marshall McLuhan, 1964 <== wow

Chapter 1: Hunters and Gatherers of Medical Information

This chapter lays the foundation for the body of the document, opening with two compelling stories of what we might today call "e-patient pioneers" – those individuals who, with no precedent, took matters into their own hands, embodying the e-patient idea that they (and you and I) have every right to know everything they can about their health – and sometimes they might even do a better job than the doctors.

Sections:

- Edward Murphy's incredible story of trying to get information about his condition – he had to impersonate his doctor (1994)

- "An unusual sloshing sound inside her head": Marian Sandmaier diagnoses her daughter's severe headaches, when two specialists had failed to (1999)

- Turning to Dr. Google: research from the Pew Center for the Internet & American Life, documenting that patient googling is now dominant: the great majority of Internet users look for medical information. (That seems obvious today, but it was radical and almost verboten when Tom Ferguson started his work.)

- Three types of e-patients – the well, the newly diagnosed, and the chronically ill – and more Pew research on the different ways they use the Internet

- "The Accepting, the Informed, the Involved, and the In Control": an intriguing way of viewing different people's Internet use based on their attitudes and how deeply in trouble they are.

In that last section, check out Group IV: "...believe in making their own medical choices... will often insist on managing their own medical tests and treatments as they think best... may attempt to help to keep their clinicians up to date on new treatments and studies.... may start, manage, or contribute to local support groups, online communities, blogs... " My my, which group am I in? :)

Chapter 2: Content, Connectivity, and Communityware – seven preliminary conclusions

This chapter was my personal favorite, because it exploded so many myths and provided so much evidence that the change is already well underway.

Remember, I didn't read this until late January 2008, six months after my treatment had ended. When I read it, my immediate question to the e-patient working group was, "How the (#@$!

could I have gone through last year without ever hearing about this?? We need to get the word out!" So here we are.

From the introduction:

> "John Seely Brown... notes that when established experts first consider the effects of new information technologies and the cultural transformations they produce, they typically do so from within the cultural constraints of their established professional paradigm ... We were no exception. Our findings were so unexpected that we were forced to consider alternative points of view... But as Brown discovered, 'Really substantive innovations – the phone, the copier, the car, the PC, the Internet – drastically alter social practices.'"

The authors – mostly doctors, remember – said "Our most helpful insights came from a growing awareness that e-patients use the Internet in three fundamentally different ways: to access content, connect with others, and collaborate with others in ways never possible before."

See what I mean about how this had strong echoes for me? They continue:

> ... many who have attempted to study or explain e-patients and many leaders in medical reform have overlooked, ignored, downplayed or even actively opposed some of the most innovative developments in modern medicine.

Presenting their findings, they said "We modestly suggest that the tentative conclusions below are no more 'anti-doctor' or 'anti-medicine' than the conclusions of Copernicus and Galileo were 'anti-astronomer.'" The preliminary conclusions:

- e-patients have become valuable contributors, and providers should recognize them as such.

- "When clinicians acknowledge and support their patients' role in self-management ... they exhibit fewer symptoms, demonstrate better outcomes, and require less professional care."

The art of empowering patients is trickier than we thought:

202

"We now know that empowering patients requires a change in their level of engagement, and in the absence of such changes, clinician-provided [information] has few, if any, positive effects."

We have underestimated patients' ability to provide useful online resources:

Fabulous story of the "best of the best" websites for mental health, as determined by a doctor in that field, without knowing who runs them. Of the sixteen sites, it turned out that 10 were produced by patients, 5 by professionals, and 1 by a bunch of artists and researchers at Xerox PARC!

We have overestimated the hazards of imperfect online health information:

This one's an eye-opener: in four years of looking for "death by googling," even with a fifty-euro bounty for each reported death(!), researchers found only one possible case.

"[But] the Institute of Medicine estimates the number of hospital deaths due to medical errors at 44,000 to 98,000 annually" ... [and other researchers suggest more than twice as many].

"We can only conclude, tentatively, that adopting the traditional passive patient role ... may be considerably more dangerous than attempting to learn about one's medical condition on the Internet."

Whenever possible, healthcare should take place on the patient's turf. (Don't create a new platform they have to visit – take yourself wherever they're already meeting online.)

Clinicians can no longer go it alone.

Another eye-popper: "Over the past century, medical information has increased exponentially ... but the capacity of the human brain has not. As Donald Lindberge, director of the National Library of Medicine, explains 'If I read and memorized two medical journal articles every night, by the end of a year I'd be 400 years behind.'"

In contrast, when you or I have a desperate medical condition, we have all the time in the world to go deep and do every bit of research we can get our hands on. Think about that. What you expect of your doctor may shift – same for your interest in "participatory medicine."

The most effective way to improve healthcare is to make it more collaborative:

"We cannot simply replace the old physician-centered model with a new patient-centered model... We must develop a new collaborative model that draws on the strengths of both systems. In the chapters that follow, we offer more suggestions on how we might accomplish this."

Chapter 3: Patient-Centered Networks: Connected Communities of Care

It's astounding how widespread e-patient behavior is, considering that hardly anyone I talk to even knows it's happening.

Internet surrogates (peer caregivers, especially women, researching for another):

"In the beginning, like most health professionals and researchers, my Pew colleagues and I assumed that patients would do their searching for themselves. So we were surprised to discover that more e-patients (81%) had gone online because a friend or family member had been diagnosed with a new illness than had searched the Net following a new diagnosis of their own (58%)."

Pew research in 2006 found 93 million Americans seeking health information for themselves, another 42 million seeking information for their parents, and more.

Helping patients & families deal with a new diagnosis: when people hear of a friend's crisis, they reach out with advice and useful information.

Patient-centered support networks – a very different entity than the better-known disease-specific communities.

I'm not in the book, but my CaringBridge friends are a perfect example. They'd get email notifications of each new post I made, and sometimes they'd forward the emails to others. In Web 2.0

terms, my support "went viral," and I got advice and support from people I'd never met or hadn't seen in decades.

- Web sites that support patient-centered online health networks: The public is now more aware of CarePages and CaringBridge . But it was a very new topic in 2006.

- Why personal online health networks have received so little attention: Most people have considered the discussions very private. Not me, baby: put me out there. :)

- Providing continuing support for the incurable: "Professional medicine is often at its worst in providing continuing comfort and care for patients facing serious illnesses that are beyond the hope of cure. In such cases, the support and care patient-centered networks of family and friends provide can be a lifeline."

- What we can learn from patient-centered networks: "Patient networks are emerging as a new medical domain within which a wide variety of individuals and groups become valuable healthcare resources. Nearly all of those involved with patient-centered networks provide their services for free, and since patient-centered networks operate independently of the formal healthcare system, they are not constrained by that system's built-in limitations, inefficiencies, and defects."

- "The importance of this form of communication should not be overlooked, since individual telephone calls and emails to a person's entire network of concerned individuals puts a huge burden on the patient or the caregiver."

The following is my observation, not taken from the published paper:

Look at how this dynamic is already disrupting where value arises in healthcare. Any student of economic earthquakes can see the signs: when a new source arises that

- adds significant value to an ecosystem

- is free

- and is not subject to the establishment's constraints,

...the convergence of forces can make for an explosive shift in everyone else's value proposition, everywhere else in the ecosystem. The White Paper doesn't say so, but having been through the gauntlet myself, and being a student of business change, the signs are clear enough for me.

Chapter 4: The Surprisingly Complex World of e-Communities

In an environment where something can be created and flourish for free, unconstrained, and where there's a need for it, it's going to evolve rapidly – becoming rich and complex, and what people want.

Reading Chapter 4 was, for me, a whirlwind tour of what happens when freely available tools get into the hands of people who are seriously motivated – on their own behalf and then with a commitment to do good for others.

But rereading this chapter now, another story surfaces for me: too often, people think "we are not worthy" compared to doctors, and that's an error. Believe me, I like doctors; they saved me, and I'm not one. But believe this too: it's a complete error not to listen to experienced patients.

- **Online support communities:** as far back as 2001, 34 million people had used the Internet for a medical or personal issue. (The Web was only seven years old then.)

- **This is Crazy! This information needs to be saved!** (1995 – the genesis of ACOR, the community that served me so well 12 years later)

- **Braintalk (1994):** An e-Patient-driven Online Educational and Support Community. "We found [early neuro patient] online support groups especially intriguing ... They offered their members more convenient, powerful, and complex information and support than any of the face-to-face groups we had seen." But those groups were on isolated servers; two doctors created Braintalk to bring them together.

- **Building from the Bottom Up.** Braintalk's founders: "Many professional efforts to develop resources for e-patients have taken the traditional 'doctor knows best' approach, providing professionally created content in a top-down manner. 'In these provider-centered systems, patients and caregivers have little or no input or control,' Lester says.

'Yet the communities we'd observed – in which patients had complete control – appeared to be doing quite well without professional assistance.' 'We decided that we would think of ourselves as architects and building contractors,' Hoch recalls, 'creating an online system in response to patient requests.'"

Please think about this: Just last month a friend of mine had a major misdiagnosis turn around completely in 8 hours, with the help of today's Braintalk members – after a hospital full of doctors had completely failed, and had then stonewalled her well-informed questions about the basis for their diagnosis.

- **Online Groups Supplement, but Don't Replace, Doctors:** "Online groups ranked significantly higher than either generalists or specialists for convenience, cost-effectiveness, emotional support, compassion/empathy, help in dealing with death and dying, medical referrals, practical coping tips, in-depth information and 'most likely to be there for me in the long run.'... Specialist physicians were rated highest for help in diagnosing a condition correctly and for help in managing a condition after diagnosis."

- **Forgotten Heroes (heroic caregivers):** "Family caregivers of those with debilitating, chronic illnesses are the most numerous – and overlooked – health workers of all. There are 27 million in the U.S. alone. They outnumber all other types of health workers combined by four to one." ... "Traditional healthcare all too often leaves friends and families out of illness care. But spouses and other caregivers have so much to offer. Online support communities don't make this mistake."

- **Putting a Human Face on Medical Information:** "Learning you have a new disease can be an earth-shattering experience. One day you're "normal" and the next you're a "patient," perhaps for life. Connecting via an online support group with others who have the same condition can be immensely comforting."

- **Special benefits for those with rare conditions:** "Patients with rare cancers are often the first example of this disease their local oncologist has ever seen. So, most doctors aren't up-to-date on the latest treatments. e-Patients can learn about the treatments currently in use at the leading treatment centers from their online communities. And they can then pass this information on to their physicians."

Week after week on ACOR, I heard of kidney cancer cases where a physician, probably overwhelmed with the explosion of medical information (see #6), were out of date. Informed patients – informed by their peers – made the difference.

Other headings in this chapter need no comment:

- e-Groups are always there (24/7/365)
- Practical Day-to-Day Illness Management Advice
- Providing continuing support for the incurable
- A godsend for those with limited access to professional care
- Keeping up on the state of the art for your condition

Please think about what it says at the top of the e-patient blog: "Health professionals can't do it alone." Neither can patients, but each can bring a lot to the table. That's why the e-patient team is talking about participatory medicine.

Chapter 5: e-Patients as Medical Researchers

The chapter tells the story of Andy Martin, the e-patient who became a clinical researcher, studying his own cancer, and became the first person ever to successfully grow his type of cancer cells in a lab.

- **From passive patients to active researchers:** "Few if any researchers had considered the possibility that patients might be able to do real medical research – conducting experiments, collecting and analyzing data, and reporting significant and valid conclusions. Not until the Internet made it possible for large groups of patients with the same health concern to share their clinical experiences did the potential role of e-patients in medical research become apparent." (Did you know it was patients, not doctors, who discovered the sexual effects of Viagra?)

- **The Life Raft Group:** a research-oriented online support community: After his wife is misdiagnosed then correctly diagnosed with a cancer that had no known treatment (GIST), a researcher starts a private group of skilled professionals who are also personally involved with the disease.

- **Bypassing the "Lethal Lag Time":** After a medical break-through occurs, it takes years (often 2-3, up to 5) for the world to hear about it – even doctors. In my view this aspect of the established peer-reviewed publication process causes harm. It's truly a lethal lag.

- **Patients can spread the word.** I see this all the time on ACOR, as patients tell each other to inform their doctors about new developments.

Note: there's nothing arrogant about doing that. Remember from Chapter 2: "Clinicians can no longer go it alone." If you want, review the full text of that section.

More astounding is something that's not in this paper: the lag from concept to putting results in practice is 17 years. (This figure is from E.A. Balas and S.A. Boren, "Managing Clinical Knowledge for Health Care Improvement", *Yearbook of Medical Informatics 2000: Patient-centered Systems.* Stuttgart, Germany: Schattauer, 2000:65–70.) Can't quite believe it? Read the steps a study has to go through.

- **Parent-initiated research on reflux:** Two mothers of children with gastroesophageal reflux disease (GERD) set out to determine whether the condition is genetically transmitted. Established researchers turned them down; they persisted, gathering more data and finding similar families. They succeeded: in 2000 JAMA published their results.

- **Jannine and Liz Cody:** Told in 1985 that nothing could be done for her newborn Liz's condition (chromosome 18 deletion which leaves patients hard of hearing and retarded), Jannine Cody studied and studied, and eventually figured out that human growth hormone might help. This led to research showing that HGH does help hearing and can bring an IQ increase of 47 points.

- **Updates (not in the EP white paper):** Liz, now 23, is attending San Antonio Community College. A few weeks ago Jannine received this year's Founder's Service award from the Genetic Alliance. During the course of all this, Jannine decided to get a doctorate in genetics, and is now an associate professor at UT San Antonio.

- **Portia Iversen Tackles Autism (1995):** "At first [they] tried to persuade autism researchers to share their DNA samples with other scientists. But the researchers weren't about to turn their hard-earned results over to their competitors. 'They had their own agenda. And it didn't always lead to getting new treatments out to the people who needed them ASAP.'

  So, they started their own tissue bank, which is now the world's largest autism gene bank. Work using this gene bank is hailed by NIH Director Elias Zerhouni as "revealing clues that will likely influence the direction of autism research for years to come."

- **Parent Expertise on PXE:** Finding that their children have a rare genetic disorder, and medical science is doing nothing for it (I guess because of its rarity), parents start a tissue bank themselves and eventually find the gene that causes the condition, which "the establishment" hadn't achieved.

  They learned that in other cases where parents had helped researchers, the researchers sometimes patented the gene that the parents helped find, thus hampering other research. So these parents patented the gene themselves, to keep any doctors from doing so. Huzzah! Whose genes are they, anyway??

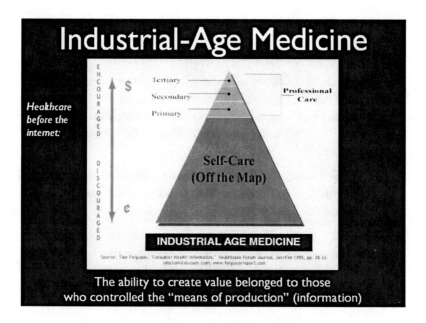

Dr. Tom Ferguson, the man who launched the e-patient movement, created these two diagrams in 1995, just months after the first popular web browser arrived. His vision of how the internet could change medicine is finally becoming reality.

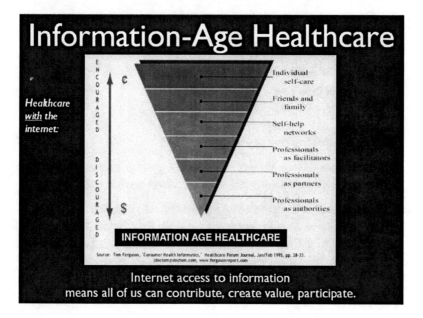

◆   ◆   ◆

Key take-aways, for me (not listed in the paper):

- The medical establishment, for all its wonderful achievements (including saving me), is nowhere near as almighty as I once thought. The careful, methodical process that we use to accumulate medical knowledge carries what can be enormous costs and penalties:

- It takes a long time for information to be developed and propagated. That makes the process very costly, which marginalizes less "popular" conditions.

- Consider Randy Pausch's testimony before Congress (see his 8-minute YouTube) about how his cancer, pancreatic, could be figured out if we had the will: he said "Let's face it," explaining his determination to make the trip and testify. "The only way you get funding is to rattle a lot of cages."

- Because of the Internet, e-patients now have the ability to connect with people around the world and become their own aggregators of information – and keep it out of the hands of professionals who would prefer to make it their own, to the detriment of the patients they're sworn to serve.

This is really starting to sound like patient empowerment, isn't it? You might want to review the two graphics on the previous page – and bear in mind that DocTom published them in 1995, when the Web was just a year old. Visionary.

Chapter 6. Learning from e-Patients

This summary is different – it's not a paragraph-by-paragraph synopsis of the primary text, it's a separate write-up of my own.

The first time I read the whole document, this chapter (the shortest in the book) lost me. It covers four distinctly different topics – it's almost odd that they're in one chapter. Lots of food for thought, but hard for me to digest. This time I dug in, and it's far deeper than its length suggests. Here's what I found:

The Internet has allowed ungoverned evolution, taking things in directions nobody anticipated. There's a lot to learn by observing what e-patients come up with when they can do anything they want.

Before the Internet, patients in need had no easy way to contact each other and satisfy their (sometimes desperate) hunger for information. The system simply was not producing what people needed and wanted. Some people died as a result, and many were unhappy or frustrated.

As previous chapters have detailed, evolution was inhibited by forces and practices in the then-current medical establishment that actively blocked lay access to information.

The Internet provides new access to information and a frictionless platform for new pathways to evolve – new ways for patients to serve each other and be served.

In this new world, things can evolve in any direction at all, without centralized planning. No authority anywhere can say No.

From an economist's point of view, a profound difference is that patients are now creating substantial value in the system with no project funding and no centralized planning. All it's required is to empower/enable people with the Internet and let them pursue what they want.

Freedom brings consequences: Patients and doctors alike have discovered that it ain't necessarily easy: pursuing the new power leads to discovering the next obstacles and challenges. New responsibility and new frustrations arise.

A new form of privacy becomes available, with new benefits: Seeking care online can provide a kind of privacy that lets people bypass their fear of stigma, so some patients are seeking (and finding) care they'd never sought before. But new responsibilities arise, and providers are evolving new practices. We learn by observing what some e-patients are drawn to when nothing's stopping them.

All that is about liberation of patient desires and energy. Sometimes we think only about how patients have been inhibited, but a potentially bigger challenge to conventional thought is this:

doctors have been frustrated too. People who think doctors are the obstacle haven't heard how hard it is to want change and be told no, by administrators and insurance clerks.

The Patient Centered Primary Care Cooperative (www.PCPCC .net) talks about how expensive and ineffective our care policies are – expensive reimbursement for specialist treatments that don't actually improve outcomes, yet inexpensive practices are vetoed, even though they've been proven helpful.

What are we to do?

That's addressed by the section on "Learning what patients really want from clinicians." It takes empowerment into a different dimension: not just treatment, but the whole relationship, and the ultimate empowerment question: Who gets to say how it's going to be?

Much of this book has been about what people do in a medical crisis – who takes action and what gets in the way. But for a moment forget about that, and just think how you'd like all medical care to work. If you could switch suppliers (as you can in many other businesses) and find any level of "customer service" and any mix of expertise-vs-self-service that you want, what would you like?

Two Harvard doctors spent two years asking patient/consumers, and this is what they found:

... insurance companies [refuse] to pay for a number of things [these patients considered] vital:

- Being available to patients by email and cell phone on a 24/7 basis.

- Giving patients access to their medical records via the Internet. This is evolving rapidly, at last – but that doesn't mean doctors are paid for maintaining the data!

- Offering newly diagnosed patients crash courses on their disorders. This lack leaves you and me to go find the information among our peers.

- Training and supporting patients to practice self-managed care. See Dr. Tom's triangles again.

- Checking clinical practices against recommended medical guidelines. Can you believe this kind of research isn't reimbursible?

- Asking patients to critique their services and to suggest better ways to meet their needs.

- Involving patients in the governance of our clinic.

- Providing online support communities for patients.

Think about that list. It would be folly in any modern business to prevent expert staff from doing what people want. Yet for the most part in America today, medical staffers can't bill insurance for those things, so they must do it "off the clock" (payment-wise) – for free.

That's what's faced today by doctors who want to use their training, their motivation, their compassion and their experience to create a new world for us. Many of us have come to accept the consequences. One doctor writes:

"Even at a world-class medical center like Boston, it's gotten so bad that most of us take the defects for granted. Patients expect long delays in getting doctor's appointments. They expect to have to wait long hours in our waiting rooms. They expect rushed, time-pressured visits from overworked, distracted clinicians. They expect to be treated rudely by clinic staffers. They expect that it will be difficult or impossible to contact their clinician in a medical emergency.

"In the traditional clinical model, the doctor essentially works for the insurance company, not the patient."

(Re letting ourselves be treated badly: Not me, you bet your bippy! When that happens to me I speak up, same as if it were a restaurant with crummy service.)

So what are doctors doing? Some are starting practices where they refuse to take insurance, and can provide exactly whatever care they want – by charging a flat all-inclusive monthly fee.

Obviously this is only for the rich – there's controversy about it. I don't have an opinion about it yet. But consider that the rich in this case (which does not include me yet!) are, in a sense, funding a form of research that's not happening anywhere else: "If you let patients have anything they ask for, what happens? Does anything new evolve?"

"The retainer-based model gives us a chance to say, 'Okay... We're really going to change things. We're going to find some exciting new ways for clinicians and patients to work together. We're going to work with our patients to develop new models of empowerment-based, patient-driven care. And if we succeed, the new practice patterns we create could provide a workable business model for widespread healthcare reform."

What's going on here? I'm not sure yet – but having worked on this post for three hours now, I'm starting to think the message is in the section title I mentioned earlier: What patients really want. We don't know yet – we're just barely starting to take off the restraints. Stay tuned, world.

♦   ♦   ♦

p.s. Two footnotes:

PCPCC's research suggests that what we really want (and certainly what employers want, as insurance buyers) is a patient-centered medical "home." When I was a kid, this was called a family doctor. PCPCC data from around the world shows that where there's good primary care, both costs and outcomes are better.

A few weeks ago Paul Levy, the CEO of Beth Israel Deaconess, commented on the money issue:

The problem with the health care "marketplace" is that it is not a real market. There are so many intermediaries that the usual connection between buyer and seller that we see in other fields does not exist. Thus, the incentives for suppliers (doctors and hospitals) to engage in efficiency improvements and value enhancement are extremely slow to emerge.

Chapter 7: The Autonomous Patient and the Reconfiguration of Medical Knowledge

> We must redefine the patient's role to emphasize autonomy, emancipation and self-reliance instead of passivity and dependence.
>
> – Angela Coulter

In some ways, it all comes down to who can make informed decisions, and "informed" comes down to who's got access to the information. That's what this chapter is about: the Internet has fundamentally changed who can get at information. (Hence, in the chapter title, "the reconfiguration of medical knowledge.")

The Internet also adds something that was never before possible: today we (patients in need) can talk to peers around the world whom we'd never have met, to share experiences and knowledge. In a complete inversion of the previous "knowledge/power pyramid," this sometimes means we the patients have access to knowledge that our doctors don't!

Think about that. Really think about it. I don't want to say "this changes everything," but it sure dynamites conventional wisdom about where to go if you want your life saved. Really think about that.

Plus, our ability to get at information and our ability to share it (and find new information from other patients) gives us an autonomy we've never had, forever freeing us from dependence on a single source of knowledge.

Ironically, this also reduces the historical burden on the physician to "know everything." That completes the profound reconfiguration of medical knowledge.

◆   ◆   ◆

Topics in this chapter:

Introduction: 3 out of 4 medical episodes are handled without a clinician, and 19/20 are partly or entirely self-managed. Only 5% are managed entirely by physicians. Could it be there's more genuine capability in lay patients than we've assumed?

The changing medical paradigm: patient web sites become the most useful sites (to patients). One researcher wrote:

"In the judgment of those who really count – e-patients themselves – the most useful online information and guidance available on a given medical topic often comes from online patients (e.g., patient webmasters and e-patient groups) rather than medical professionals.

"It is these e-patients themselves – and not their clinicians – who choose the online resources they prefer. And it is they who decide when and how to use them.

Who's in charge here, anyway? The stark contrast between the past's closed access to medical info and how that's been exploded by the Internet.

The configuration of medical knowledge in [last century] medicine: Some of the items in this section will pop your eyes open. Personally, I realized that these nasty tidbits are one consequence of not having access to the knowledge, so we had to go through a closed society to get it. We don't have to, anymore.

The only limit, frankly, is how many of us know it's happened, and have access to the Internet (no small issue, to much of the planet's population).

The pitfalls of paternalism: "Patients were considered incapable of understanding and taking charge of medical matters. ... The model for most health care is still 'doctor knows best'... The problem with this template, apart from its essentially authoritarian nature, is that the doctor may, indeed, not know best. ... Example: It took 60 years to establish that, for many patients, a simple mastectomy is just as good as a radical one."

Think about that, too, if you still feel an M.D. degree guarantees greater wisdom.

And if we can't be sure MDs know best, where can we turn? That's the point: we turn to ourselves to be responsible.

We do consult our physicians, but we also gather what info we can, and we check with our peers to see how different approaches have turned out.

Bottom line, we decide for ourselves which resources are most valuable.

Sometimes it is indeed our doctors. (That's how my peers steered me to my oncologist.) Sometimes it's elsewhere.

The e-patient-resistant clinician: A brief section: "We have used this term to identify those health professionals who refuse to acknowledge their patients' competence or to accept their influence."

Here's a recent example from May 2008: responding to a blog post on CNN, Carol K said when she asked her doctor about a treatment, he responded "Who's got the degree here?" (btw, his diagnosis turned out to be completely wrong.)

Moving beyond medical paternalism: "Coulter proposes that patients be treated as '…responsible adults, capable of gathering and assimilating information and of learning the skills needed to provide much of their own medical care.' The clinicians' roles in 21st century healthcare will increasingly be to support their patients' own initiatives, to encourage patients to practice self-managed care, to help patients acquire the information, skills, tools, and support they need, and to serve as advisors along the way." You may want to again review "Steal These Slides."

The e-patient-receptive clinician: "When patients [can] collaborate with a non-paternalistic clinician, asking questions in their own way and communicating via e-mail when needed, actual consultation times typically do not increase. Patients are more satisfied and feel that they have spent more time with their doctors – even though, in some cases, they may spend less time interacting face-to-face."

I know this from first-hand experience: when I've communicated with my providers before a meeting, so the agenda is pre-set, I always leave the meeting satisfied. And it gives them a chance to be more prepared.

Clinician Support for the Expert Patient:

"Kate Lorig and her colleagues at the Stanford Patient Education Research Center were the first to identify and study the expert patient. They found that, compared with other patients, expert patients did a much better job of managing their diseases – improving their health status, coping more effectively with fatigue, remaining less dependent on professional care, and managing the many other challenges of their chronic condition."

"Anecdotal impressions so far suggest a level of commitment and enthusiasm from patients, healthcare professionals, and managers that will carry the management of chronic disease into a new era of optimism and opportunity." Liam Donaldson, chief medical officer of Britain's National Health Service, commenting on the NHS's Expert Patient Program.

How e-Patients Can Help Healthcare: "Autonomous patients will educate themselves about their medical conditions and will manage more of their own medical care. In so doing, they will operate at a higher level:

- setting and implementing their own healthcare agendas whenever possible;

- diagnosing and treating more of their own medical conditions;

- obtaining more tests and treatments on their own;

- storing, organizing, and updating their medical information in more comprehensive and useful ways;

- preparing themselves for their interactions with medical professionals."

Patient-Initiated Quality Improvement Project: The story of a patient feedback form developed by e-patient founder Tom Ferguson MD, while he himself was a patient.

Conclusions: "As Coulter warns, clinicians must accept patients as partners. If they do not, the healthcare system will be vulnerable to a widespread loss of confidence. But if they do, there is the potential for more patients to help themselves to the health care that they need."

◆　　◆　　◆

I think it's fitting to end by repeating what I said at the start of this chapter:

In some ways, it all comes down to who can make informed decisions, and "informed" comes down to who's got access to the information. That's what this chapter is about: the Internet has fundamentally changed who can get at information. (Hence, in the chapter title, "the reconfiguration of medical knowledge.")

The Internet also adds something that was never before possible: today we (patients in need) can talk to peers around the world whom we'd never have met, to share experiences and knowledge. In a complete inversion of the previous "knowledge/power pyramid," this sometimes means we the patients have access to knowledge that our doctors don't!

Think about that. Really think about it. I don't want to say "this changes everything," but it sure dynamites conventional wisdom about where to go if you want your life saved. Really think about that.

Plus, our ability to get at information and our ability to share it (and find new information from other patients) gives us an autonomy we've never had, forever freeing us from dependence on a single source of knowledge.

Ironically, this also reduces the historical burden on the physician to "know everything." And that completes the profound reconfiguration of medical knowledge.

◆   ◆   ◆

I know I've read something that alters my view when I can return to the beginning and find that it has a whole new meaning. Here's the quote that opened Chapter 1 of this white paper:

> "[People] are suddenly nomadic gatherers of knowledge...
> informed as never before...
> involved in the social process as never before...
> [as] we extend our central nervous system globally..."
>
> — Marshall McLuhan, 1964

Don't you just love a visionary?

Appendix B
Thoughts on Statistics
and Medical Evidence

When my crisis was over and my learning about e-patient began, I kept bumping into something that causes policies, patients and even providers to be severely misinformed: misuse of statistics.

For e-patients, caregivers, and policy makers, this is important enough that I devoted a whole chapter to it earlier, and still had enough left over for this appendix. If you'd like to play a more active role in medical decision-making, understanding what treatment is being recommended and why, you'll find this section useful. Leading doctors and scientists who've reviewed this have said I'm right – we ordinary citizens are capable of understanding more about this subject than we might think, and we should indeed do so.

I'm no statistical genius but I learned enough in school to understand the basics: you need to understand what people were looking at when they drew their conclusions. Plus, serious statisticians have a wide range of measures available, and it's important not to use the wrong one, or you'll accidentally reach a bad conclusion – just as bad as if a map didn't tell you a bridge is out.

As you'll see in the blog posts below, that's a problem when you're making public policy, and it can really be a problem when you're making decisions about your health.

Saturday, December 8, 2007

For prettier statistics, omit inconvenient people

The two top rantables on my agenda right now are statistics and silos. This time it's statistics. I'm irked because I keep seeing a mistake that blows the kneecaps off any well-intentioned effort to improve policy by looking at statistics. People need to be aware of it, spot it, and cry "BS!" when it rears its head.

Earlier this week, in Paul Levy's blog I got into a discussion in the comments section of a post. Frequent and knowledgeable contributor Barry Carol had wondered if high healthcare spending around here might be caused in part by a large supply of hospital beds and specialists locally. I said, in part:

I'm intrigued with Barry's observation. (I don't have an opinion – I don't know the data he cites; I'm just intrigued.) Is it accurate to say the cause is too many beds? Or is it that more are available, so it's possible to give someone the care they need? (I then recounted a story of my father's care in his final decade, where the hospital staff only seemed to become competent when it was time to kick him out.)

If motorists were spending lots of money on fixing flats, would we say the problem is that we have so many tire repair shops? It's not a perfect analogy, but it's worth looking at. Some cultures think women are the cause of rape, because if there weren't all those women, there wouldn't be all those rapes.

I feel strongly that any statistics about costs and outcomes in a system should have an accountant's note specifying what proportion of the population goes without coverage in that system, so they don't even have an outcome. Until we get honest about that, all we're doing is chasing a bubble under the blanket.

There's the rub, the itchy spot. In cases like this, the goal of statistical analysis is to better understand things, particularly to know what a batch of data does or doesn't represent so we can predict the best way to approach future situations. And if we don't know what those statistics left out, we don't know what we'd be getting ourselves into by relying on them. We cannot rely on findings until we know what cases were and weren't included.

Increasingly, what might be getting omitted is you. Or someone you love.

As the boomers age, and their decades of productivity and home buying convert to decades of home selling and health costs (who, me?), this is gonna be a big skull-knocking issue. There will be claims about which system works better, with all kinds of statistics being flung around like monkey dung. (Sorry, but monkeys do fling dung when they're fighting, and when policymakers start fighting, they fling statistics, claiming they're proving reality.)

For health policy, all kinds of claims can be made with good statistical support – but you better ask who got left out, making the picture prettier, whether it was intentional or not.

Overlooking the inconvenient people isn't limited to healthcare costs. Consider the following, from the US Dept of Labor's Bureau of Labor Statistics (BLS):

- Unemployment statistics don't include everyone who wants a job but can't find one. Once your unemployment benefits run out, they simply stop counting you. You don't even exist as a problem anymore, as far as the BLS is concerned. I cannot figure out a legitimate reason for this.

- There are no statistics for people who eventually gave up on their previous career and are now working for half their previous pay. People in that situation are, again, simply not counted as a concern.

- Nor are there statistics for the loss of benefits. Employers certainly pay less for no-benefit or feeble-benefit jobs, but if you or I change to a job with no benefits, it doesn't even make a dent in the pretty statistics.

- Worst of all, the "jobs created" statistics are a cruel joke. When a full-time job with benefits is carved up into three part-time jobs with no benefits, the BLS counts it as job growth. (I called my Senator's office and had them check it out; a senior BLS statistician got back to me and confirmed it.)

This is insane. It's as if King Solomon chopped up 1,000 babies and declared a population explosion.

What is wrong with these people?? In May of 2006 an erudite observer in the New York Times remarked with surprise about the 200,000 "new jobs" that had been created in April: "employment [is] doing well, yet core inflation has remained remarkably subdued." Remarkable indeed, until you know what they're calling "job creation."

As I say, until we get honest about this, all we're doing is chasing a bubble around under the blanket. With the best intentions, we'll make misguided policy decisions. And believe you me, policy has impact at the personal level. The time will come when you (or a loved one) is the bubble everyone wants to chase away. Do whatever you can to stop this crap. Now. Wake up! And wake others up.

Saturday, November 15, 2008

Making sense of health statistics

This was a pivotal moment: discussion on our blog revealed that policy people, politicians, reporters and even doctors commonly misinterpret numbers they've read. As you'll see, the resulting errors are entirely understandable by lay people; we need to look into the conclusions.

John Grohol, Psy.D., is founder and publisher of PsychCentral, a pioneering community of e-patients. After he read my post the other day about evidence-based medicine, he sent me a paper worth reading: "Helping Doctors and Patients Make Sense of Health Statistics." (To read it, Google "Make Sense of Health Statistics".)

This is relevant to the e-patient movement because as you and I become more responsible for our own healthcare, we need to be clearer about what we're reading. Plus, it appears we could be more vigilant about what our own professional policymakers are thinking.

The paper is 44 pages, longish, but even the first few will open your eyes to how statistically illiterate most of us are – and that includes MDs.

Consider this question, which was given to 160 gynecologists. Assume the following information about the women in a region:

- The probability that a woman has breast cancer is 1%.

- If a woman has breast cancer, the probability that she tests positive is 90%.

- If a woman does not have breast cancer, the probability that she nevertheless tests positive is 9% (false-positive rate).

A woman tests positive. She wants to know whether that means that she has breast cancer for sure, or what the chances are. What is the best answer?

1. The probability that she has breast cancer is about 81%.

2. Out of 10 women with a positive mammogram, about 9 have breast cancer.

3. Out of 10 women with a positive mammogram, about 1 has breast cancer.

4. The probability that she has breast cancer is about 1%.

21% of them got the right answer (#3, 1 chance in 10). 60% guessed way too high, the other 19% guessed #4. (That's 10 times too low.)

The paper presents numerous other examples of statistical illiteracy (an example of "innumeracy"), misunderstandings of data that lead to serious unintended policy consequences. My personal favorite is the opening item about Rudy Giuliani's assertion that he's lucky to have gotten prostate cancer here instead of under the UK's "socialized" medical system. It's not because I don't like Giuliani – it's that his own misunderstanding of the data he was quoting led him to advocate something that had nothing to do with his actual odds. He himself would have been harmed if he'd been guided by his own best advice. And he's not alone in that.

The paper proposes uncomplicated ways to improve our comprehension. First among them is to stop talking in percentages and talk instead in raw numbers. Phrased that way, the same three facts that were given to the gynecologists is much clearer:

- Ten out of every 1,000 women have breast cancer.

- Of these ten women with breast cancer, 9 test positive.

- Of the 990 without breast cancer, 89 nevertheless test positive.

- With this view, 87% got it right. (Of the 98 women who tested positive, only 9 actually have cancer: about 1 in 10.)

Another example echoed what *The End of Medicine* said about Lipitor. (Without Lipitor, 1.5% of the control group had a coronary event; with Lipitor, about 1% still had one.) A 1995 alert in the UK warned that certain oral contraceptives doubled the risk of blood clots in the lung or leg. Understandably, many women stopped taking the pill; within three years, 13,000 more abortions were performed, reversing five years of decline, and there was a matching increase in live births.

What was the risk that led to this? In raw numbers, one woman in 7,000 has such a blood clot anyway; with this pill, one more blood clot happened.

The irony in this case is that both abortion and childbirth carry more risk of clots than the pill itself. In other words, one benefit of the pill is that it avoids the risk of clots associated with the end of any pregnancy.

So although the number presented ("double the risk") was absolutely accurate, the real clinical impact wasn't nearly as absolute.

This is a taste of what's in the first few pages. It gets dry in places but even the first few pages are compelling and informative – and at no point does it require that you be a mathematician. The explanation of Giuliani's error is particularly good.

Saturday, November 22, 2008

More on statistics: deadly omissions, deadly conflicts

Dr. Ted Eytan pointed out a great website that evaluates the quality of health news reporting, HealthNewsReview.org.

Gilles Frydman, founder of ACOR, dug into it and wrote a post at the e-patients blog called "Lies, Damn Lies And Statistics: Collective Statistical Illiteracy".

Gilles continued Thursday, partially inspired by the issues raised by HealthNewsReview, and wrote the slash-and-burn post "No other conflict of interest, huh?" He pastes in the conflict of interest fine print that appears at the end of the article: 345 words of disclosures about how the article's authors receive funds from the makers of the medications described in the article. The disclosure ends with this delightful phrase: "No other potential conflict of interest relevant to this article was reported."

And this was no tabloid rag – this is in the *New England Journal of Medicine*, one of the most respected journals in the world.

What would you think about news reporting by writers who are literally being paid by the people they're reporting on?

I think I'm going to make a point of keeping an eye on HealthNewsReview, and maybe start bitching at the NY Times when I spot them omitting vital information like that.

Anyway: in the comments on that post, Sarah Greene, who recently left the NY Times online health department, speaks from the perspective of someone who's been on the inside of a big modern news organization. In her comment she remarks, "More to the point, patients don't get to wear that E-badge if they aren't first Educated to understand Evidence."

She adds, "My shock-disbelief-sadness centers on the media. Can journalists be held accountable at a time when news organizations are pushing for more & faster & shorter, coupled with desperation for digital advertising dollars?"

All in all, I agree with Sarah's remark that it's up to you and me to dig into the numbers when a treatment is recommended. As the "Make Sense" paper says, if we don't know the actual numbers, the whole concept of "informed consent" doesn't work.

And, sadly, a new contributor, Karen Vaughan, speaks up from the diabetes community and highlights something I hadn't noticed about the NEJM study mentioned above: "About 20% more people got diabetes in the drug group. For every life 'saved' by the drug, someone else got diabetes. Factor that into the 'costs' of the drug." That issue too is reported in the "Make Sense" paper:

every treatment (or decision not to treat) has side effects, and no informed choice is possible unless all that is laid out.

Vaughan answers the balance question, concluding: "If a person took a 30 minute walk per day they would have better results without the side effects or costs."

Wouldn't you think those alternatives should be laid out for our consideration in a journal that purports to inform the medical trade about how best to achieve health? I don't mind reporting on new medications, but simple decent scientific method requires documenting all the known, relevant pro's and cons.

Appendix C
Finding Online Support Groups

This sidebar was suggested (and authored) by Jan Alexander, wife of publisher George Alexander, as she read the manuscript. I couldn't agree more.

When I was diagnosed with bladder cancer, it was my second cancer diagnosis in two years. A year earlier, I had been diagnosed with breast cancer, and I joined several online support groups. But I never really engaged with them. My breast cancer was found early, and had a non-controversial treatment path. In addition, I found a wonderful in-person support group at the hospital where I had my surgery that gave me the emotional support I needed during those early traumatic days after diagnosis.

My bladder cancer experience was entirely different. I had no knowledge whatsoever of the disease, and had never known anyone who had it. I felt alone and terrified. I went to Google to learn something about bladder cancer, and my search results immediately pulled up posts from an online support community discussing the very issues I was concerned about. I went to the site and joined, an act that saved my sanity at the time. It was enormously helpful to find people in my situation who had made it through what I was going through, and were generous in sharing their support and knowledge.

That was only one of four bladder cancer groups I eventually joined (each for a different reason). What follows is some wisdom I gained from my experiences.

Different groups have different styles. Each disease will have multiple online support groups, and they will vary in sponsorship. In addition, they will vary in format (some posts will arrive as regular email, others are a community you can join that allows you to post pictures, write blogs or journals, etc.). These factors will make a difference in the character of the group.

I found during the early traumatic stage right after my diagnosis that I needed not just practical advice, but also a tremendous amount of emotional support. One forum I joined was excellent for offering top notch advice. Another I found excellent for providing emotional support, because it offered the opportunity for people to post their pictures, write in their journals, send private messages to each other, and let me know in my email when someone had replied to a discussion I had started. I formed close ties with some of the people because I had seen a picture of what they looked like, had corresponded with them privately, and even ended up talking with several of them by phone.

Now that I am through that awful period right after diagnosis, I am finding a different site extremely useful, because several of its members keep us up to date on the latest treatments and research, and many people post what they are doing to try to prevent their cancer from returning.

So, my advice is to lurk for a little while when you first find a group, and see if you like the tone of the posts you are reading. Post a few trial questions and see how people respond. You will gradually get a feel for the nature of the group, and know if you want to continue with it or not. Avoid like the plague groups that are just people commiserating about their illness, but instead, look for empowered, engaged and proactive patients who are taking charge of their own health. They will help keep you going through some very difficult times, and will be the source of invaluable advice.

Check on who is sponsoring the site, and whether there are medical professionals who contribute their expertise to the forum. Find out if the group is run by people who actually have the disease, and find out what the parameters for posting are. All these things may make a difference in the usefulness of the group for your needs.

Suggestions for finding a group. Start with these umbrella organizations that host online support groups:

ACOR (Association of Cancer Online Resources, www.acor.org) provides access to over 150 mailing lists that "provide support, information, and community to everyone affected by cancer and related disorders".

INSPIRE (www.inspire.com) hosts hundreds of online health related support groups, including over 50 support groups related to cancer.

MedHelp (www.MedHelp.org) is an online community with eight million members including professional medical advisors.

Major Cancer Societies. Check out the websites of major cancer societies for your disease, as they often host their own online support groups.

These are a few initial ideas for finding groups, and they have worked well for me. But there are many other groups out there (some wonderful and some not so good). Ask everyone you can find, including your doctors and fellow patients, to recommend their favorites.

— Jan Alexander

Acknowledgments

In 2007 while sick I kept a journal at CaringBridge.org, where family and friends could read the latest news and leave supportive notes. This book is largely distilled from those entries, which might make it sound easy. But it took a lot of work: the journal was many times longer, and the book adds blog posts about things I learned later. A lot of work.

In a moment I'll repeat my 2008 thanks to the clinicians, e-patients and CaringBridge "fans" who were with me through my Stage IV cancer. But first I want to thank the people who turned the journal into the book.

◆   ◆   ◆

I've known my publisher **George Alexander** for decades, since I was a young product manager in typesetting and he was perhaps the best analyst in my industry. When George Alexander wrote something in The Seybold Report on Typesetting Systems, about my own product or a competitor's, I knew it was well researched and carefully reasoned. He taught me how to think about the production process.

I've crossed paths with George several times, most recently last fall, when he met me at an e-patient conference and said, "I think there's a book in your story." I agreed: "Yeah, everybody says that. But I don't have time to do it." He replied, "I'll do it." Long story short, here we are: his small publishing company Changing Outlook Press has produced this book in less than a year.

George had the vision for the nature of this book: episodes from my journal plus subsequent learnings. He did the work, plowing through nearly everything I've ever posted and stitching pieces together. He did such a great job that I myself was amazed at the story when I read it!

George is wise, gentle, astute, competent, and sensitive. This is Changing Outlook's sixth book, and if there's justice in the world they'll have great success in their future endeavors.

I want to thank, also, several people who taught me the skills that fuel my presentations and my best blog posts.

Dorron Levy, my best friend, appears many times in the story. Dorron taught me the most sacred of lecturing skills: how to arouse a deep curiosity in an audience, so that they're gripped with the question "How can this be??" When that question is satisfied, people's minds change, and sometimes their lives change.

Dorron is also the smartest person I know: he digs deep, deep, deep into the fundamental questions of why things are the way they are, which helps understand what changes will make any difference. I believe his thoughts about health data can change what medicine looks like in the future. We should ask his advice about everything.

Thom Hartmann, a longtime mentor, taught me several pivotal things: the power of online communities, the power of how we choose to view things (including matters of well-being), and how to be responsible for a classroom or audience. He and his wife Louise are co-founders of the New England Salem Children's Village and The Hunter School, superb facilities for children with ADHD, Asperger's and related conditions. I've been a board member with Thom for more than ten years. They do difficult work, but that's never stopped Thom.

George Carlisle was the first mentor in my career. Born a few days after me, George shot past me as we both worked in the typesetting industry. He was the first to teach me persuasion: how to write and speak such that a complex idea reveals itself. And during my illness he generously served as one of the "Davey-Sitters" described in the book.

Several people contributed invaluable advice and feedback on specific sections:

- **Peter Schmidt** gave a rigorous review of the statistics sections, substantially improving them.

- Members of my ACOR kidney cancer community gave feedback on the chapter on Facing Death – With Hope:

Janet Curtis, Dave Dobbins, Matt Ivy, Sandy Massie, Larry Mulligan, Tammy Russo, Jill Siebers, Terry Wilson.

- Proofreading and editorial reviews were offered by **Mom** and **Stephen Edwards**.

- And now, it's time to repeat my acknowledgements – still heartfelt years later – for the people who stood by me at the time, and who lit the path I follow today in spreading the word about e-patients: "Empowered, engaged, equipped, and enabled."

Acknowledgements from my original online journal

When I first published my unabridged journal, here's what I included.

Contributors to my CaringBridge journal

Wife Ginny, amazing singer-sister Suede, Mom, all of Suede's phenomenal and powerful supporters (especially Jere, Leslie and Sallie), my high school and college classmates, my professional friends and colleagues, and everyone else who posted. You have no idea how much of a difference you made. It was an incredible experience to see you keep popping up. (Please, readers, do not fail to offer words of support to others. It matters.)

Contributors to my care

- Ginny, Sandy, Mom, and the "Davey-Sitters": Matt Mercier, John Englander, Jeff Evans (all members of my chorus), and Sally Jensen. And Ginny, again and again.

- **Beth Israel Deaconess Medical Center**, especially Dr. David McDermott, Kendra Bradley RN, MeeYoung Lee NP, Virginia Seery NP, orthopedist Dr. Megan Anderson, and Dr. Drew Wagner. And CEO Paul Levy. If you care about health care, please follow his blog.

Laugh, Sing, and Eat Like a Pig

The e-patients movement

I'd never heard of the e-patient movement until January 2008, yet e-patient principles and practices were present throughout the book's conversations. As I learned a year later (January 23, 2008), "e-Patients are those that use email and the internet to become empowered to manage their own health and become partners with their providers."

E-Patient Resources (though I didn't know it at the time):

• The PatientSite patient portal at Beth Israel Deaconess.

• ACOR.org, host of the KIDNEY-ONC email group that gave me the fastest, most up-to-date information about my condition and answers to my questions at the times when I needed them most. Unlike any other source of Internet information, my ACOR peers were unfailingly reliable and available. Special thanks to Gilles Frydman, founder of ACOR and member of the e-Patient Scholars Working Group.

• www.CaringBridge.org, host of the discussions reproduced in this book. (You can see my brief video testimonial on YouTube.)

Harvard Pilgrim Health Care. We hear a lot these days about what's wrong with health care, especially insurance companies. If I'd had a bad insurance company it could have added significant stress to my situation; instead I had a great one. Particular praise to Helen McNabb, my cancer care coordinator.

The Nashua Granite Statesmen men's barbershop chorus. They're the "sing" in this book's title. This group provided a type of support I could never have imagined. I hesitate to single out any one individual at the cost of not naming others, but I give special thanks to then-director Steve Tramack and performance coach (now director) Jim Coates.

Landmark Education, creator of the courses and additional graduate training that taught me about empowerment, or, as they put it, "freedom, power, and full self-expression." Many people have expressed amazement at how I handled that year. I say, if you want to see who you really are, you might try giving up who you've been being, and Landmark is the handiest, most readily available vehicle I know for achieving that.

And, of course, I acknowledge the one and only **Dr. Danny Sands**, my primary care physician, co creator of PatientSite, a compassionate man and member of the e-Patient Scholars Working Group. Most of all, Dr. Sands has always trusted me to be his partner (not his subordinate) in managing my care – a fundamental tenet of the e-Patient movement. Little did I know how much I was getting when I took him as my doctor.

I hope you can sense how deeply, deeply grateful I feel – blessed, even – to have benefitted from so many wonderful people. Thank you, all, then and now.

Index

CPSIA information can be obtained at www.ICGtesting.com
Printed in the USA
BVOW05s2354290315

393856BV00030B/803/P

9 780981 650432